Hatha Yoga

MANUAL TWO
by Saṁskṛti and Judith Franks

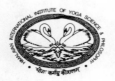

Published by

Himalayan International Institute
Honesdale, Pennsylvania

ISBN 0-89389-043-X

Copyright 1978
Second Pringint 1979

Himalayan International Institute of Yoga Science and Philosophy
RD 1, Box 88, Honesdale, Pennsylvania 18431

Dedicated to our reverend teacher
Shri Swami Rama of the Himalayas
from whom we have been learning.

The authors would like to express a special thanks to the following people whose work was invaluable in bringing this book to print: Dr. Agnihotri—for checking the Sanskrit terms, Doug Bill—postures, Gary Evers—photography, Theresa O'Brien—typesetting the manuscript, Randy Padorr-Black—cover design, and Janet Zima—layout.

Contents

ॐ सहनाववतु । सह नौ भुनक्तु ।
सह वीर्यं करवावहै ।
तेजस्विनावधीतमस्तु । मा विद्विषावहै ।
ॐ शान्ति: । शान्ति: ॥ शान्ति ॥।

PRAYER OF HARMONY
 For Teacher and Student

OM Sahana Vavatu
Sahanau Bhunaktu
Sahaviryam Karavavahai
Tejasvinavadhitamastu
Ma Vidvishavahai
OM Shantih Shantih Shantih

Oh God, Protect us both together,
Accept us both together,
Let us achieve strength,
Let our learning ever shine,
Let us not resent each other.
OM   Peace Peace Peace

Introduction

The *Hatha Yoga Manual II* is designed to help the continuing student become aware of the more subtle aspects of yoga. While beginners may start the practice of yoga purely for its physical benefits, the finer dimensions of hatha soon present themselves. Though physical mastery of the *asanas* can come quite quickly, mental prowess in their performance may develop over years.

In the *Hathayogapradipika* it is stated, "Neither can Hatha Yoga be perfected without Raja Yoga, nor Raja Yoga without Hatha Yoga." We see that yoga practice is designed as a continuum—so hatha yoga must be understood as far more than physical exercise.

In yoga the body is considered to be a gross manifestation of the mind. One's mental state may be observed in the way that one "carries oneself,"—but not only are one's thoughts reflected through one's posture, one's posture also shapes one's present character of mind.

Careful observation of the experience of yoga *asanas* will lead one to notice a change in one's "mental posture." Hatha yoga loosens those bonds of habit by which one has mentally restricted the body, and reinforces the "mental flexibility" which one already enjoys. One begins to consciously limber the body only to find that a corresponding sense of freedom is unfolding in the mind.

Thus hatha yoga is an intensely personal experience. One's progress is not judged by the degree to which one stretches, but rather by the manner in which the postures are performed.

Persistent practice will lead to a stronger body and a vitalized mind, and truly provides the means for greater self-understanding. It was with these ideas in mind that this manual was written, and to this end it is hoped they will find their expression.

Matthew Monsein, M.D.
May 10, 1978

Who Should Use This Manual?

This manual is the second in a series of texts which follows a systematic program of hatha yoga courses developed by the Himalayan Institute Teachers Association in the tradition of H. H. Swami Rama. It is designed for those students who have successfully mastered the postures, breathing, and relaxation exercises in the *Hatha Yoga Manual I*. It can also serve as a useful text for those students who have been following other traditions of hatha yoga *if* the methods of practice as outlined in the beginning manual are studied and practiced for some time. It is therefore important that before using this text *all* students again carefully read the sections in the *Hatha Yoga Manual I* on Attitudes, Hints, and Cautions, Yama and Niyama, and Diaphragmatic Breathing.

At the intermediate level a student of hatha yoga should be firmly established in his practice. Daily repetition of the postures becomes increasingly important as more difficult postures and their variations are attempted. Gradually the postures should be perfected, preparatory exercises eliminated, and new postures added to one's daily routine. This is also the state of development at which students should become increasingly aware of the subtle effects that postures have on the body, breath, and mind. This process can be facilitated by asking oneself questions such as:

How does this particular posture affect my body?

How does it affect my mind?

What is happening to my breath?

How is my breathing affecting the postures?

Am I concentrating on the posture or is my mind wandering?

Am I releasing or creating tension in the posture?

Am I relaxing those parts of my body which are not directly affected by the posture?

Always take a few minutes to relax, be quiet, and center your mind before beginning your practice. After this the basic sequence of postures to be followed is:

1

Limbering
Standing Postures
Meditative and Sitting Postures
Backward Bending Postures
Forward Bending Postures
Inverted Postures
Twisting Postures
Headstand
Relaxation
Breathing Exercises

Many of the postures (i.e., cobra, locust, bow) from the *Hatha Yoga Manual I* are not repeated in this text. This does not mean, however, that these postures should be eliminated from one's daily routine of practice.

The asanas within this text have been grouped as much as possible in the above categories. The meditative asanas, however, are not considered cultural asanas, and as such comprise a separate section (V). The balance asanas are not grouped together, but are disbursed in those categories in which they most appropriately fit. Within the cultural asana section are also included a number of exercises which either prepare you for advanced postures or increase flexibility in specific parts of the body. Only those postures which are considered part of traditional hatha yoga bear Sanskrit names.

The preliminary steps shown in this manual are important in order to perfect the postures; master them before adding the advanced variations. It is as important in this manual as in the beginners manual to read all the instructions, including the preliminary exercises, cautions, and benefits before attempting a posture. And again, be sure and review all the instructions for practice outlined in the *Hatha Yoga Manual I*. Remember that no manual on a practical subject, such as hatha yoga, can substitute for studying with a qualified teacher. If you are practicing on your own, exercise care and common sense at all times.

For deeper understanding of the subject of hatha yoga, three texts are recommended in conjunction with this manual: *Lectures on Yoga*, by Swami Rama, *Philosophy of Hatha Yoga* by Usharbudh Arya, Ph.D. and *Science Studies Yoga* by James Funderburk, Ph.D.

2

SHAT KRIYAS

SHAT KRIYAS/Purificatory Exercises

In the intermediate and advanced practice of hatha yoga great stress is laid upon not only the external, but also the internal cleanliness and purification of the physical body. The *kriyas* or purificatory exercises help eliminate excess mucus, toxins, and impurities from the body. The word "kriya" means action or act, and in this context refers to cleansing activity. The *shat* (six) *kriyas* commonly known to yogis are:

1) *dhauti*
2) *basti*
3) *neti*
4) *trataka*
5) *nauli*
6) *kapalabhati*

These exercises are means of cleaning the throat and esophagus of excess phlegm, keeping the stomach free of excess acid, the bowels of feces and gas, and the lungs, pores, and sweat glands free from waste and impurities. Chapter II, verse 21 of the *Hathayogapradipika* explains who should practice the *kriyas*: "One who is flabby and phlegmatic should first (before the practice of *Pranayama*) practice the six acts. Others (who do not have these defects) should not practice them, the (three) humours (wind, bile, and phlegm) being equally balanced in them."

The result of this practice is explained in verse 23: "These six cherished processes, which purify the body and yield wonderful results, are held in high esteem by the foremost of yogis." Of the *shat kriyas*, *neti, trataka,* and *kapalabhati* can be practiced by intermediate students of hatha yoga. Instructions for their correct practice are given in this and the *pranayama* sections. *Nauli* can be practiced by advanced students, whereas *dhauti* and *basti* should be practiced only under the supervision of an experienced, qualified instructor.

4

(1) **Dhauti** is the name given to a number of methods for cleaning various internal organs.

   (a) *Vastra dhauti*—cloth dhauti. A fine muslin cloth three or four inches wide and twenty-two and one-half feet in length is swallowed and then drawn out again. This cleans and massages the mucus membranes of the throat, esophagus, and stomach.

   (b) *Brahma-datuwan dhauti*—similar to *vastra dhauti*, except that a bent stick or rope is used instead of a cloth.

   (c) *Kunjar kriya*—upper wash. A large quantity of water is drunk and then vomited out.

   (d) *Prakshalanam*—complete wash. A large quantity of water is drunk and then, through the use of specific exercises, expelled through the rectum.

   (e) *Vayu-prakshalanam*—swallowing air and forcing it out the bowels. Another process of swallowing air and then belching is not recommended by experts because it can create gastric problems. Whereas in *vayu-prakshalanam*, if there is a problem or hindrance the exercise can be safely completed with the help of several postures, such as *pavan-muktasana*.

   (f) *Ganesh kriya*—cleaning the rectum.

   There are also *dhautis* for cleaning the mouth, throat, and teeth.

(2) **Basti**—cleaning the colon. This *dhauti* is similar to an enema; water is drawn into the colon, held, and then released. In *basti*, unlike an enema, water is not forced into the colon, but drawn into the intestines when a partial vacuum is created by exercises and mudras, such as *nauli* and *aswini mudra*.

(3) **Neti**—cleaning the nasal passages. There are two methods of doing this:
   (a) *Jala* or water neti
   (b) *Sutra* or string neti
   In *jala neti* water is used to clean the nostrils by taking it from nostril to nostril, nostril to mouth, or mouth to nostril. A small china pot with a narrow spout, called a "neti pot," can be used for this process (see photo).

Technique
   Fill neti pot with warm (not hot) water and add just enough salt (without

5

iodine) so that you can taste it. Either too little or too much salt will cause irritation of the mucus membranes lining the nose. Practice this exercise over a sink or basin. Three methods of *jala neti* are explained below. When the first method has been mastered, the student can practice the other two methods.

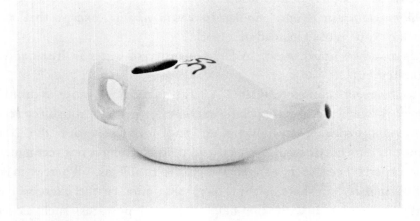

(1) **Nostril to Nostril**

Insert (gently) neti pot into the active nostril. (Description of active and passive nostrils has been given in Pranayama section of *Hatha Yoga Manual I*). If the spout of the neti pot is too large to fit into the nostril, place it so that it covers the nostril. Tilt the head to the side until it is nearly parallel to the ground. Let the water run in the active nostril and out the passive. If the water does not come out of the passive nostril or runs down the cheek, simply adjust the tilt of the head. The water should flow in a smooth, steady stream.

(2) **Nostril to Mouth**

a. This may be done at the same time as side to side neti if the head is at the proper angle. Tilt the head sideways as in the first exercise, but with forehead raised. Relax the throat and let the water drain into the mouth.

b. Nostril to mouth neti can also be done by putting the neti pot at the nostril and then tilting the head back. Be careful not to allow the water to go down the throat; it should be expelled through the mouth. The student should use whichever of these methods is easiest for him.

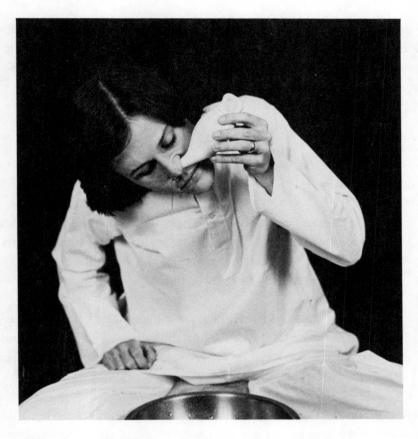

JALA NETI—NOSTRIL TO NOSTRIL

(3) Mouth to Nostril

Put salt water into the mouth. Bend at the hips and flex the neck, bringing the chin toward the chest. Make slow, partial swallowing movements of the throat muscles while relaxing the soft palate (tissue between the nasal cavity to the mouth). Let the water drain from one nostril. Take more water and drain it out the opposite nostril. Finally, let the water drain through both nostrils simultaneously. The nostril from which the water drains depends on the tilt of the head. This method should be attempted only after the other two have been mastered. It is not difficult but it does take more practice to place the head in the proper position and perfect the swallowing movement which forces the water from the mouth out the nostrils.

7

After *jala neti*, blow both nostrils using a quick, forceful exhalation. Then use the hands to close alternate nostrils, and exhale more gently. If for some reason water accumulates in the sinuses, any or all of the following exercises may be used.

1. *Trikonasana* (Triangle). See page 72 of *Hatha Yoga Manual I* and page 42 of *Hatha Yoga Manual II.*

2. Side to Side *Kapalabhati.* See Pranayama section, page 158 of *Hatha Yoga Manual II.*

3. Position yourself on hands and knees with the back straight. Exhaling, rotate the head and look over the right shoulder. Inhaling, turn the head back to center. Exhaling, look over the opposite shoulder. Inhaling, turn back to center. Repeat three times.

4. Assume the child's posture (*Balasana*, page 122 of *Hatha Yoga Manual I*) with the head resting on the floor. Inhaling, raise the hips and roll forward from the forehead to the crown of the head. Exhaling, come back. Repeat slowly three times.

(4) **Nauli**—isolation and rolling of the *rectus abdominus* muscles. *Agnisara* is not technically considered a *kriya*, but is a very useful preparatory exercise of *nauli*. *Agnisara* is explained in detail in the *asana* section of this book.

(5) **Trataka**—gazing exercise. *Trataka* can be practiced in the morning after relaxation and before *pranayama*. There are two points of concentration: *brumadhya drishti*, the point between the eyebrows, and *nasagra drishti*, the tip of the nose. Concentrate the gaze on either of these two points and hold for as long as comfortable. Relax the eyes. If the eyes become red, sore, or tear, hold for a shorter length of time. Maximum 20 seconds.

Benefits

Increases concentration, strengthens the eyes.

(6) **Kapalabhati**—cleaning the respiratory organs. This is explained in detail in the pranayama section of this book.

8

BANDHAS & MUDRAS

Bandhas and Mudras

Mudra means "to seal"; any action that seals the strength of man is *mudra*. It also means "short," a short cut to yoga, because *mudras* are a help and means to various accomplishments in yoga, particularly during the initial steps of breathing exercises. There are twenty-five *mudras* and *bandhas* mentioned in the *Gheranda Samhita.** Those which are useful for students at this stage are explained below. More difficult ones should only be attempted under the guidance of an expert.

* One of the traditional hatha yoga texts.

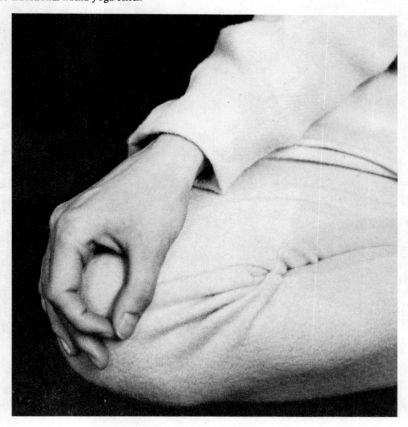

JNANA MUDRA

11

(1) *Jnana* or *chinmudra*—symbol of knowledge. Place the thumb and forefinger together and then rest the hands comfortably on the knees. This *mudra* is used for *pranayama* and meditation.

(2) *Vishnu mudra*— Fold the index finger and the middle finger of the right hand. The thumb is used to close the right nostril and the ring finger is used to close the left nostril. This mudra is used for (during) *pranayama*.

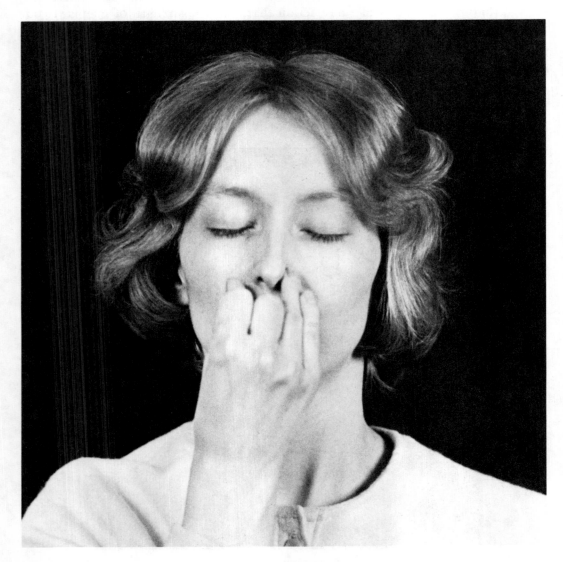

VISHNU MUDRA

12

(3) *Aswini mudra*—Horse *mudra*. Pull the buttocks in and contract the anal sphincter muscles. Hold for 2-3 seconds, then relax. Repeat 7-10 times. Practice standing and then sitting in the easy posture. *Aswini mudra* prepares one for practicing *mulabandha*. This *mudra* is also helpful for people suffering from constipation or hemorrhoids.

(4) *Yoga mudra*—Symbol of yoga. See asana section.

Bandha means "to close, to stop, to bind, to lock." These *bandhas* are used during *pranayama*, concentration, and meditation. Their use during specific exercises will be explained in those sections. The *bandhas* should not be used with the asanas unless specified.

(1) *Jalandhara bandha*—Chin lock. Bend the head forward and press the chin against the chest, as well into the jugular notch as possible. This *bandha* gently pulls on the spine. It is used during certain *pranayama* exercises.

(2) *Mulabandha*—Root lock. This *bandha* is similar to *aswini mudra*, in that the anal sphincter muscles are contracted. However, in *mulabandha* both the external and internal sphincter muscles are contracted and then held. This *bandha* is used during *pranayama* and meditation.

(3) *Jihva bandha*—Tongue lock. Curl the tongue up and back as far as possible toward the soft palate. Keep the tongue in this position during *pranayama* and meditation.

(4) *Uddiyana bandha*—Stomach lift. See *Hatha Yoga Manual I.*

13

MEDITATIVE ĀSANAS

Meditative Āsanas

Asanas are of two types—cultural and meditative. While there are at least eighty-four cultural *asanas* with thousands of variations, the main meditative *asanas* are only four: *sukhasana*—the easy posture, *padmasana*—the lotus posture, *siddhasana*—the accomplished posture, and *swastikasana*—the auspicious posture.

In the *Yoga Sutras*, Patanjali defines asana as "a particular posture of the body, which is steady and comfortable." (Sadhana pada, sutra 46.) He is referring not to the cultural postures but to the meditative *asanas* which are used during *pranayama* (breathing exercises), *dharana* (concentration) and *dhyana* (meditation).

In all of the meditative *asanas* great emphasis is placed on keeping the head, neck, and trunk straight. "The posture is perfected, made steady, and comfortable through relaxing, not forcing the effort and by fixing the consciousness on the Infinite."

The erectness of the meditative postures can be checked as follows:
(1) Assume any one of the four meditative postures.
(2) Place the hands on the thighs, palms downward with the fingers pointing toward the hips and the heel of the hands next to the knees. Keep the elbows straight. (See photo.)

In this position the spine is completely straight. Maintain this same erectness whenever using the meditative posture. Once a posture is chosen it should not be changed again and again. Rather, be constant and practice that particular posture until it is perfected.

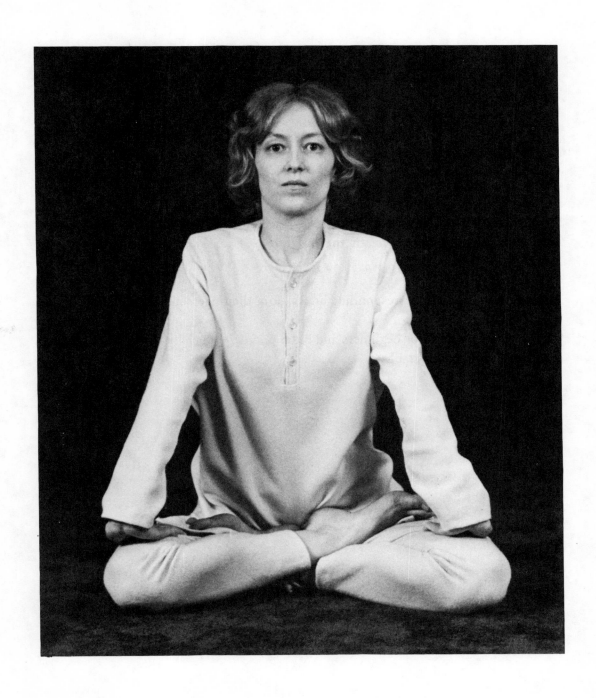

17

SUKHĀSANA/Easy Posture

This is a simple cross-legged posture.

Sit with the head, neck, and trunk straight. Place the left foot beneath the right knee and the right foot beneath the left knee. Each knee rests on the opposite foot.

Place the hands on the corresponding knees; join the fingers in *jnana mudra*.

This posture is useful for beginners and older people, especially if the other postures are painful or uncomfortable.

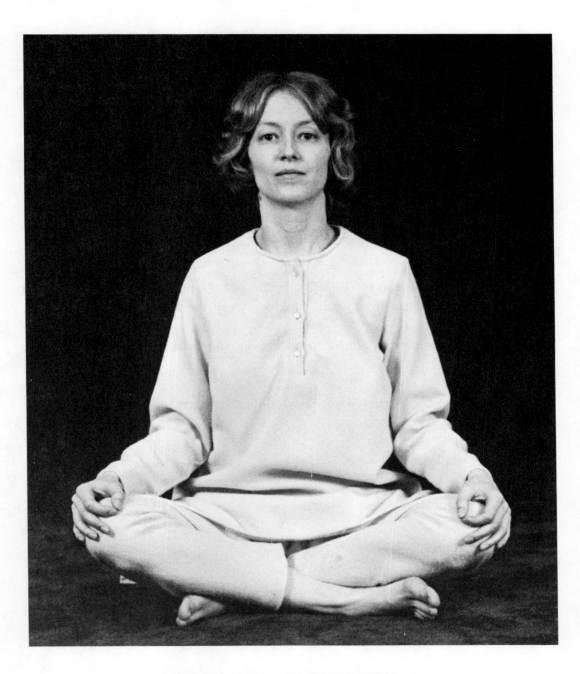

SUKHASANA — EASY POSTURE

19

SWASTIKĀSANA/Auspicious Posture

This posture is similar to *Siddhasana* except that the heels and ankle bones are not aligned.

Bend the left leg at the knee and place the sole of the left foot against the right thigh.

Place the right foot on top of the left calf and put the outer edge of the foot and the toes between the thigh and calf muscles. Only the big toe should be visible.

Then, pull the toes of the left foot up between the right thigh and calf so that the big toe is visible.

Place the hands on the corresponding knees; join the fingers in *jnana mudra*.

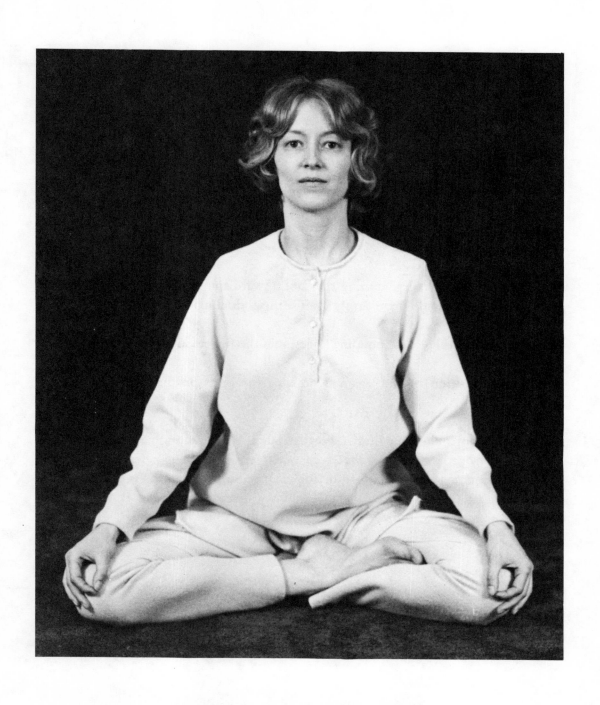

SWASTIKASANA—AUSPICIOUS POSTURE

21

PADMĀSANA/Lotus Posture

Sit with the head, neck, and trunk straight, extend the legs in front of the body.

Bend the left leg and take hold of the foot turning up the sole. Place the foot firmly at the right groin.

Similarly fold the right leg, turning the foot upward and placing it firmly at the left groin. Both heels should press firmly against the abdominal wall.

Place the hands on the corresponding knees; join the fingers in *jnana mudra*.

Reverse the position of the legs and practice the lotus posture with the left leg on top.

Padmasana is not only a meditative posture but is also used in many *asanas* such as *matsyasana, yoga mudra, bandha padmasana,* etc. Some experts contend that *padmasana* is not a desirable posture for meditation because it is very difficult to do *mulabandha* (contraction of the anal sphincter muscles) in this posture. If, however, *padmasana* is used for meditation, the right leg should be on top.

22

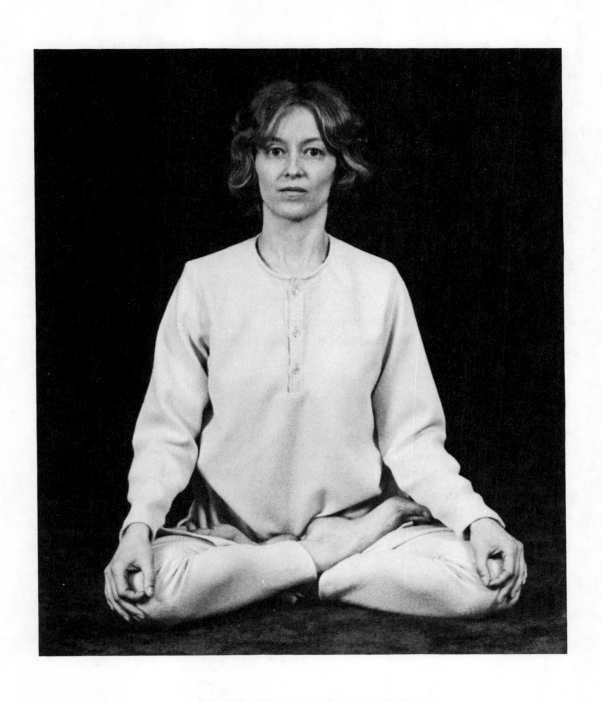

PADMASANA—LOTUS POSTURE

23

SIDDHĀSANA/Accomplished Posture

Sit with the head, neck, and trunk straight.

Apply *mulabandha* (root lock) and then place the left heel at the perineum (region between anus and genitals). Place the right heel at the pubic bone above the organ of generation. Arrange the feet and legs so that the ankles are in one line or touch each other.

Place the toes of the right foot between the left thigh and calf so that only the big toe is visible. Similarly, pull the toes of the left foot up between the right thigh and calf so that the big toe is visible.

Place the hands on the corresponding knees; join the fingers in *jnana mudra*.

Siddhasana is considered by adepts to be the best posture for meditation. Because of the pressure exerted by the heels on the genitals, the benefits from this posture are greater for men than women. *Siddhasana* is helpful in the practice of continence and celibacy. The benefits of *swastikasana*, the auspicious posture, are similar to *siddhasana* and this posture is highly recommended for women.

24

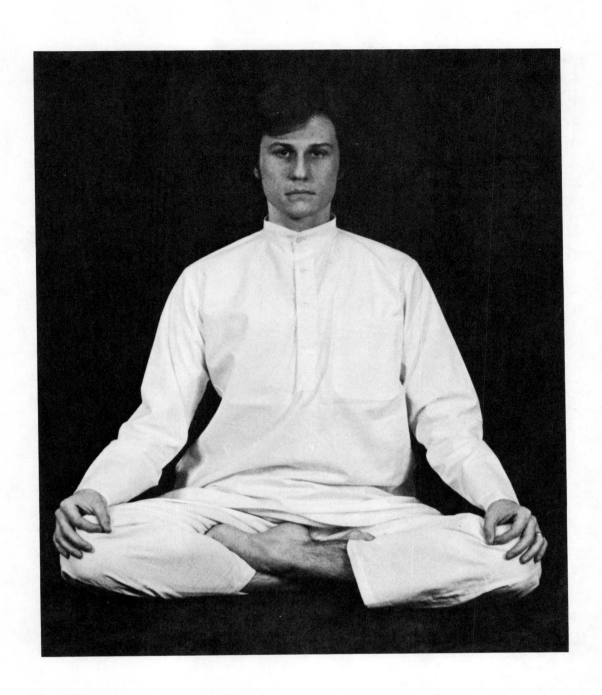

SIDDHASANA—ACCOMPLISHED POSTURE

HERO
SERIES

Hero Series

Although not considered part of traditional yoga postures by many schools of hatha yoga, the hero series, like *soorya namaskara*, is an excellent warm-up exercise; it stretches and limbers the spine and limbs.

Practice 1-3 rounds. The hero series is more strenuous than the sun salutation so the student should increase the number of rounds very slowly. Its benefits and guidelines for practice are the same as those outlined for the sun salutation (see page 42 of *Hatha Yoga Manual I*).

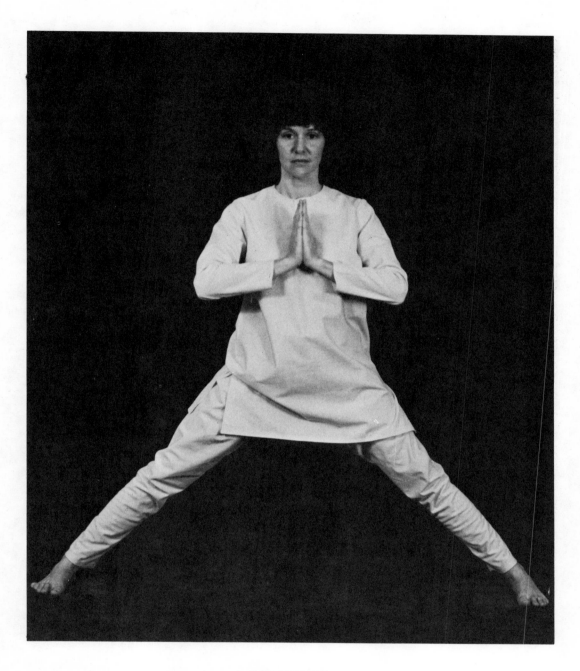

POSITION 1

Stand firmly with the head, neck, and trunk in a straight line; the feet should be as far apart as possible. Place the palms together in prayer position at the chest and gently close the eyes. Standing silently, concentrate on the breath for a few seconds.

29

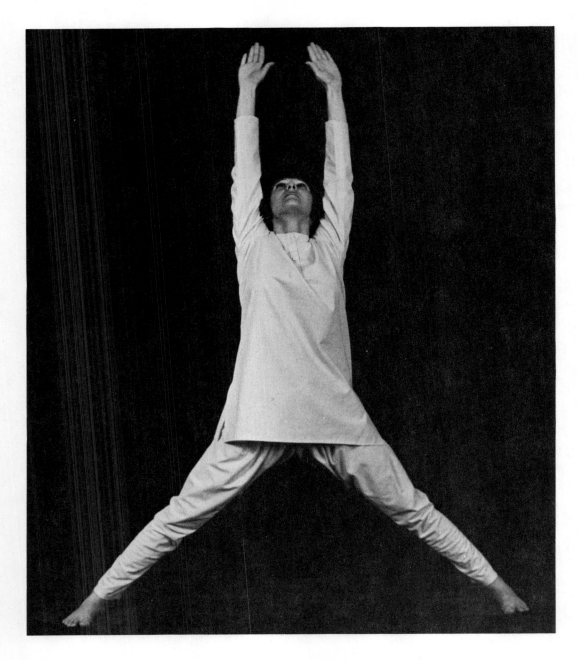

POSITION 2
Raise the arms above the head, look up, and begin to bend back.

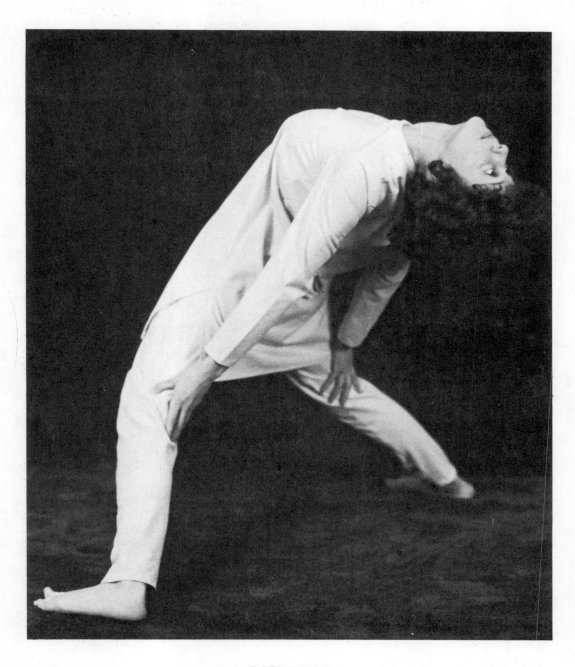

POSITION 3

Bend back as far as possible sliding the hands down the thighs.

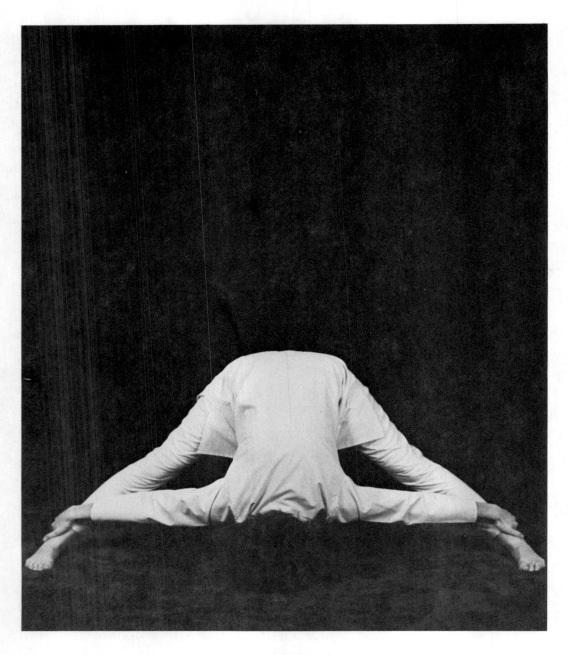

POSITION 4
Bend forward and continue to slide the hands down the legs to the ankles.

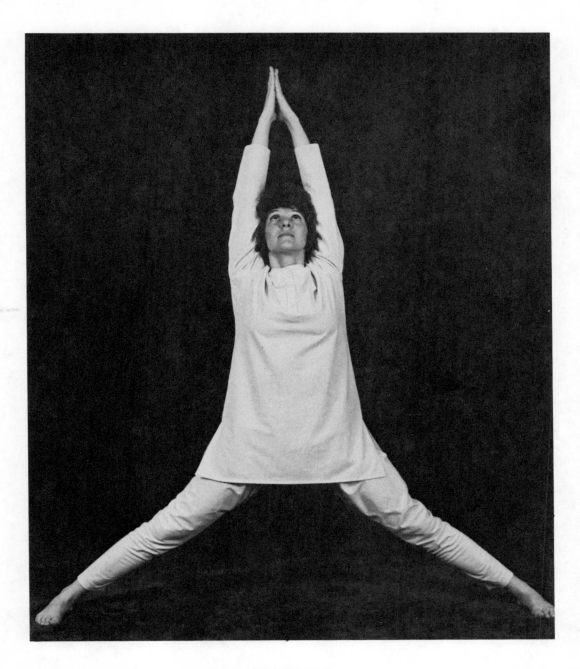

POSITION 5

In the forward bend, bring the hands back to the chest in prayer position and slowly raise. Keeping the hands in the prayer position, raise the arms above the head.

33

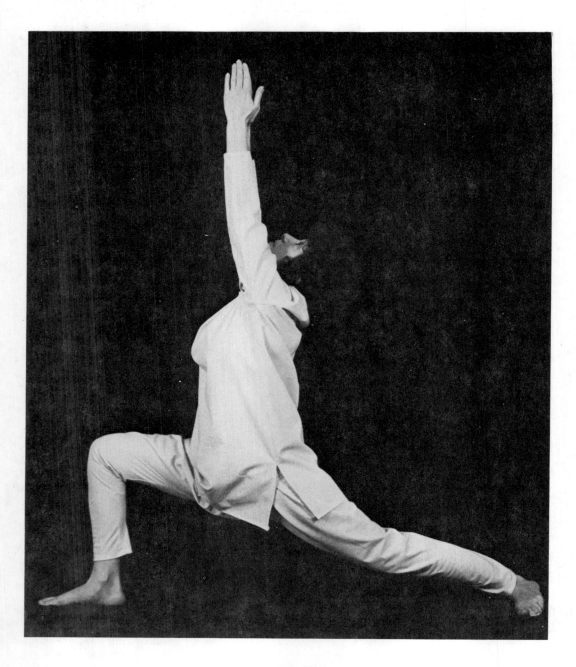

POSITION 6
Turn the right foot 90°. Turn the body to the right. Bend at the right knee and lower the thigh until it is parallel to the floor. The lower leg and thigh form a right angle. Look at the palms.

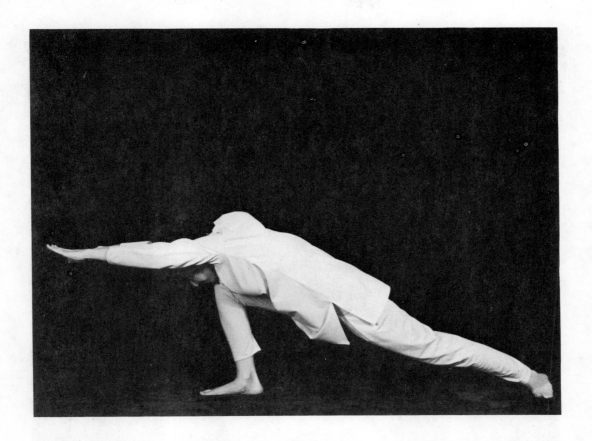

POSITION 7
Keep the arms and legs in the same position and bend from the waist until the chest touches the upper thigh. The arms are extended and the palms may either remain in prayer position or face downward.

POSITION 8
Keep the right thigh parallel to the floor, raise the torso, turn the head upward and look at the palms (same as Position 6).

POSITION 9
Straighten the right leg and turn the body and foot to the front. The arms remain above the head in prayer position (same as Position 5).

Repeat steps 6-9 on the left side.

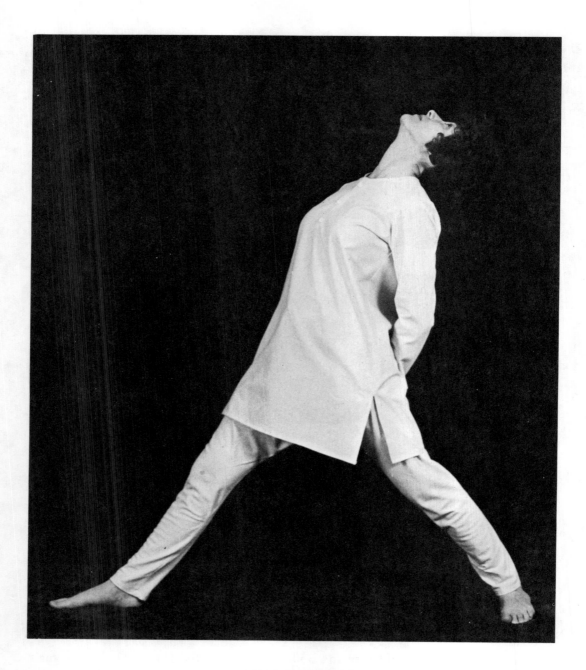

POSITION 10

Lower the arms, place them behind the back and grasp the right wrist with the left hand. Keep the heels in line and place the right foot at a 90° angle from the left. Turn the body to the right and bend back as far as possible.

36

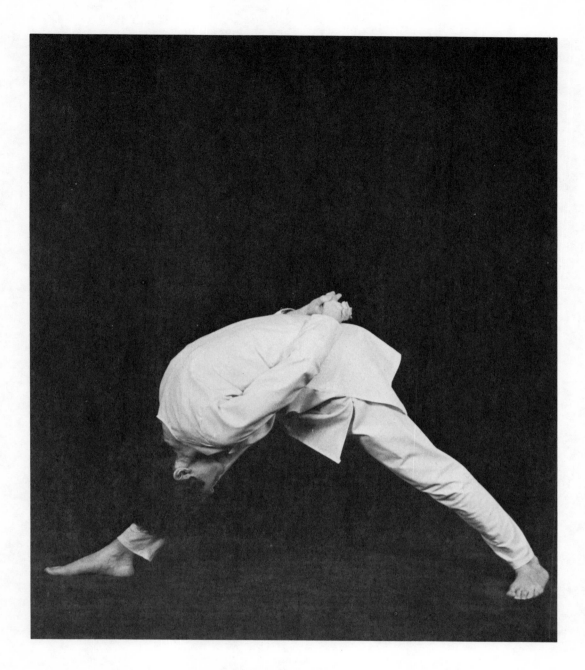

POSITION 11
Bend forward from the hips and bring the head to the right knee.

37

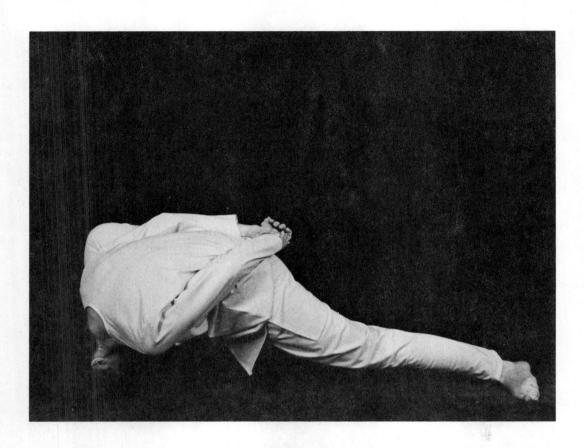

POSITION 12
Bend the right knee. Then continue to bend from the hips until the forehead touches the floor inside the right foot.

POSITION 13
Raise the body and turn the torso and foot back to the front.

Repeat positions 10-13 on the left side.

38

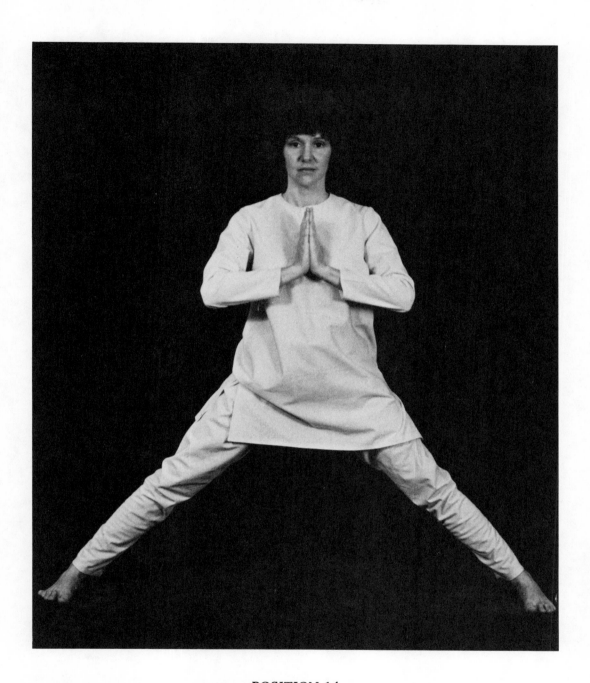

POSITION 14

Complete the series by bringing the hands back to the chest in prayer position, gently closing the eyes, and concentrating on the breath for a few seconds. Then, relax completely.

39

CULTURAL
ĀSANAS

TRIKONĀSANA/Triangle

Variation 1

Stand with the head, neck, and trunk in a straight line, legs three feet apart. Inhaling, slowly raise the arms to shoulder level with the palms facing downward.

Twist the trunk to the right. Exhaling, bring the left hand to the inside of the right foot, keeping the arms and the legs straight. The arms remain in line with each other, and the right arm extends straight up. Look up and back at the right hand.

Breathe evenly; hold for 20 seconds.

Inhaling, slowly return to a standing position.

Repeat, bringing the right hand to the inside of the left foot.

Variation 2

Repeat the posture as described above turning the foot at a 90° angle. Place the hand on the floor at the inside of the foot.

Variation 3

(See photo.) Repeat the posture as described in Variation 1 and place the hand on the floor at the outside of the foot.

42

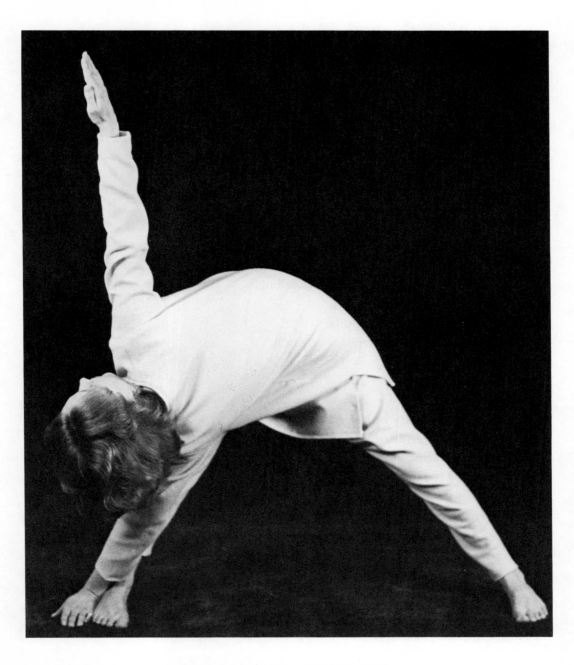

TRIKONASANA—TRIANGLE
Variation 3

Variation 4
(See photo.) Repeat the posture as described in Variation 2 and place the hand on the floor at the outside of the foot.

Variation 5
(See photo.) Stand with the legs as far apart as possible. Turn the right foot at a 90° angle.

Inhaling, raise both arms and then slowly bend the right knee until the thigh is parallel to the floor.

Exhaling, bring the left arm next to the ear and bend sideways and place the right hand at the inside of the right foot. The left arm is parallel to the floor with the palm turned downward. Look up at the ceiling.

Breathe evenly; hold for 20 seconds.
Inhaling, slowly return to a standing position.
Repeat on the opposite side.

Benefits
　　　Increases flexibility of the spinal column and hip joints
　　　Lengthens the hamstring muscles on the back of the thigh
　　　Variation 5 also:
　　　Stretches the muscles and ligaments of the pelvis
　　　Stretches all the muscles along the side of the torso, arms, and legs.
　　　Strengthens the arms and shoulders

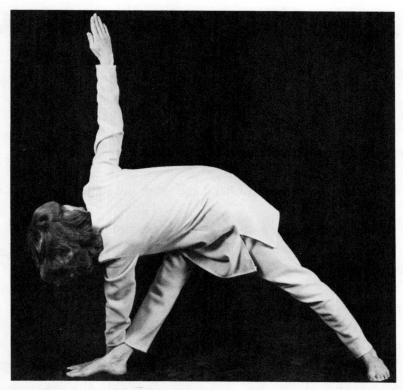

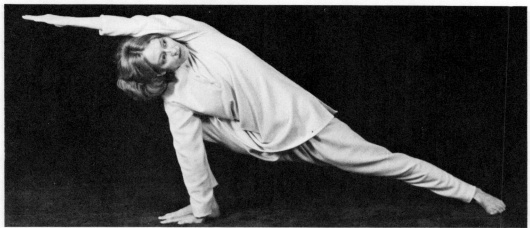

TRIKONASANA—TRIANGLE
Variations 4 and 5

45

ARDHA-BANDHA VRIKSHĀSANA
Half Bound Tree

Stand in the tree posture with the right foot in half lotus.

Reach behind the back with the right hand and grasp the foot.

Extend the left arm forward keeping it parallel to the floor.

Breathe evenly; hold for 30 seconds.

Repeat on the opposite side.

Benefits
- Develops poise, concentration, and balance which is helpful for the performance of all postures
- Increases flexibility of the hips, knees, and ankles

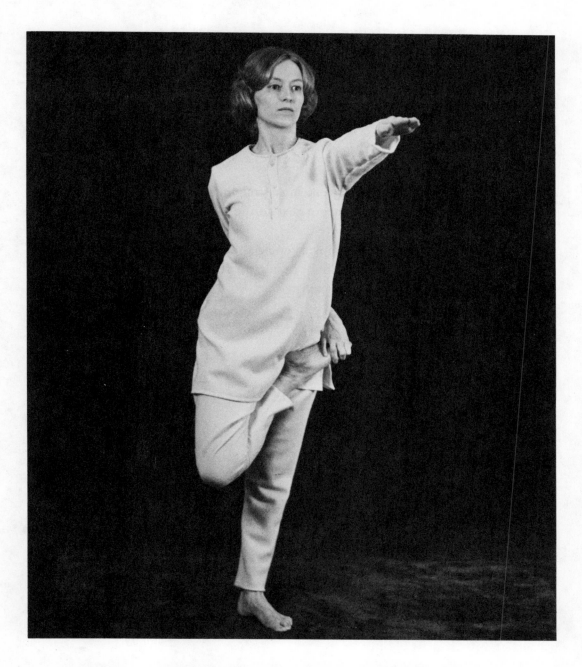

ARDHA-BANDHA VRIKSHASANA—HALF BOUND TREE

PADAHASTĀSANA
Hand~to~Foot Posture

Variation 1
Stand with the head, neck, and trunk in a straight line, feet together. Inhaling, stretch the arms overhead until they are next to the ears.

Exhaling, bend forward from the hips, keeping the back straight and the arms next to the ears; place the hands on the floor beside the feet, with the fingers next to the heels and the heels of the hands next to the toes.

Keep the legs straight and pull the chest toward the legs.
Breathe evenly; hold for 20-30 seconds.

Inhaling, raise and relax.

Variation 2
(See photo.) Repeat the posture as described above, except this time place both hands beneath the feet.

Breathe evenly; hold for 20-30 seconds.

Benefits
- Same benefits as in the sitting forward bend (see page 116 of *Hatha Yoga Manual I*)
- Relieves constipation
- Decreases excess abdominal fat
- Makes the spine supple and stretches the hamstring muscles

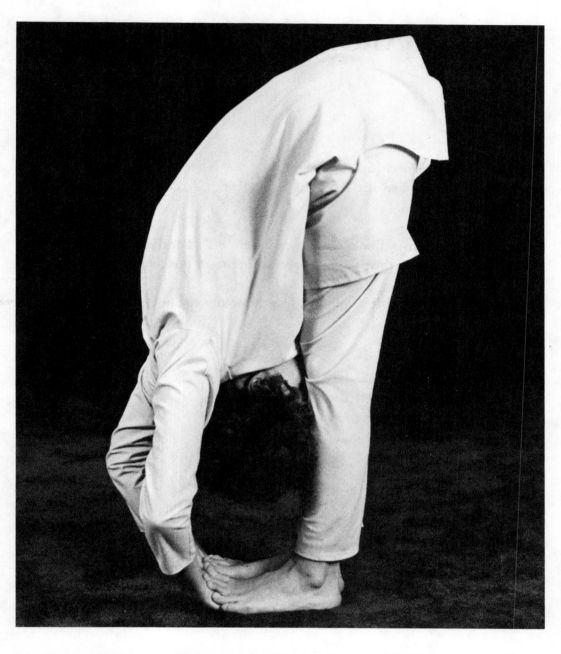

PADAHASTASANA—HAND-TO-FOOT POSTURE
Variation 2

49

GARUDĀSANA/Eagle

Stand with the head, neck, and trunk straight.

Bend the left knee, then lift the right leg and wrap it completely around the left leg (see photo).

Cross the right arm over the left arm forming an "X." Continue wrapping the arms around each other until the palms are together in prayer position.

Gaze at a point slightly above eye level, breathe evenly and hold for 30 seconds.

Repeat on the opposite side.

Benefits
- Develops poise, concentration, and balance
- Strengthens the ankles and legs
- Increases flexibility of shoulders, arms and wrists.

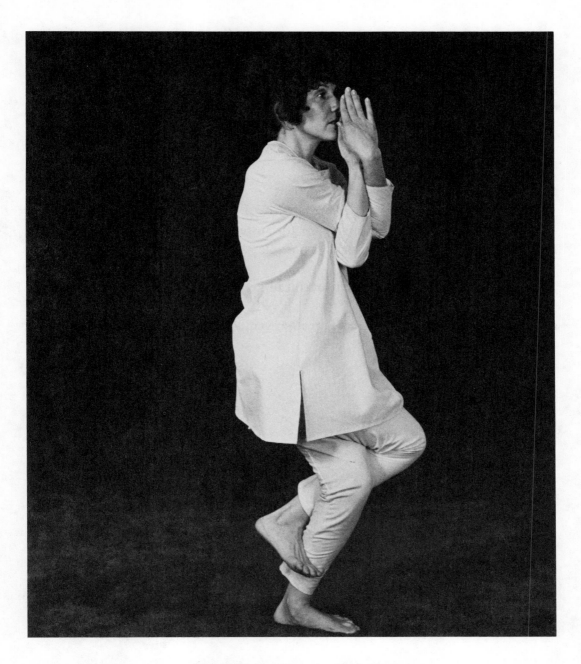

GARUDASANA—EAGLE POSTURE

51

Preparation for
NATARĀJĀSANA/King Dancer

Position 1
Stand with the head, neck, and trunk straight.

Exhaling, bend the left knee and grasp the instep of the foot with the left hand. Pull the foot as close to the buttocks as possible.

Inhaling, lift the right arm straight overhead keeping the arm in line with the ear.

Gaze at a fixed point straight ahead, breathe evenly and hold for 10-20 seconds.

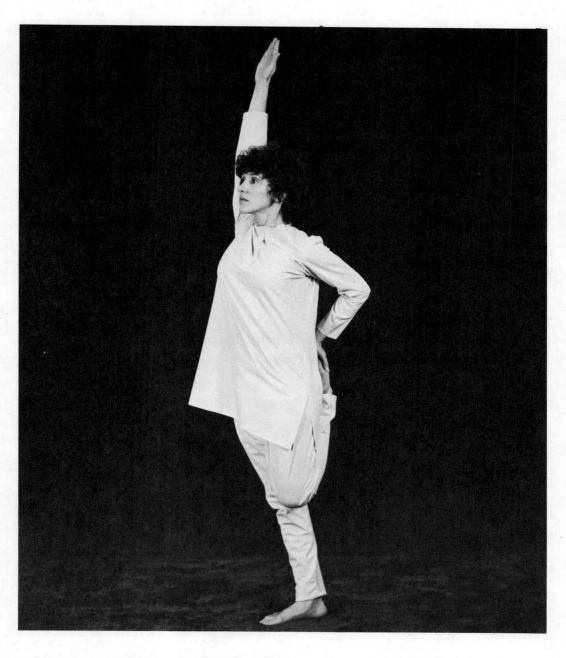

PREPARATION FOR *NATARAJASANA*—KING DANCER
Position 1

Position 2
Continue from Position 1 into Position 2.

Exhaling, bend from the hips without bending the spine and tilt the upper torso forward.

Inhaling, and keeping a firm hold on the instep of the left foot, lift the leg until the thigh is parallel to the floor. Expand the chest and gently pull the shoulder blades closer together.

Gaze at a fixed point straight ahead, breathe evenly, and hold for 10-20 seconds.

Repeat both positions on the opposite side.

Benefits
    Expands the chest
    Releases tightness and stretches the pelvic ligaments
    Develops poise, balance, and concentration

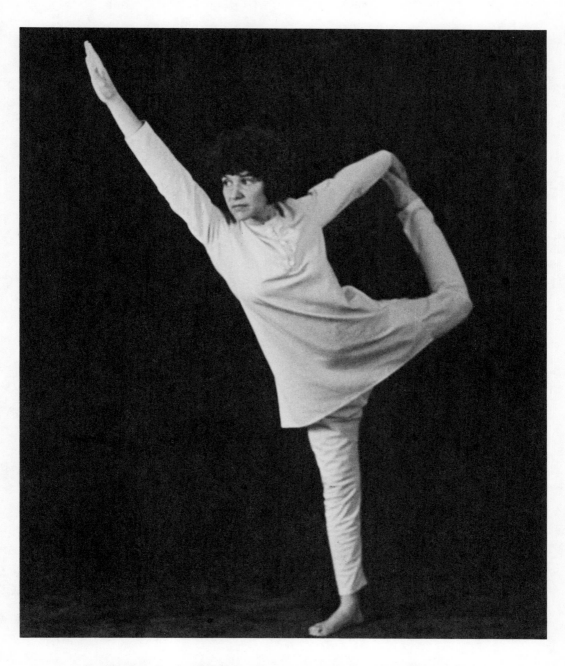

PREPARATION FOR *NATARAJASANA*—KING DANCER
Position 2

55

VIRĀSANA/Warrior Posture

Position 1
Sit in a kneeling position with the knees together and feet beside the body so that the buttocks rest on the floor. Keep the head, neck, and trunk straight.

Breathe evenly; hold for 30 seconds.

Position 2
Keeping the knees together, turn the feet outward so that the toes point away from the body.

Breathe evenly; hold for 30 seconds.

SUPTA VIRĀSANA
Reclining Warrior Posture

Sit in position 1 of *virasana*. Gently lean back until the body rests on the floor. Fold the arms above the head.

Breathe evenly; hold for 30 seconds.

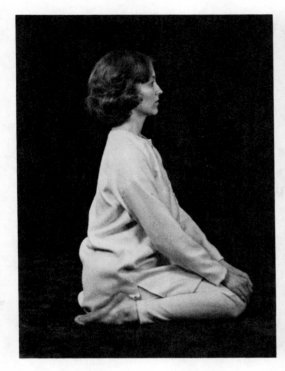 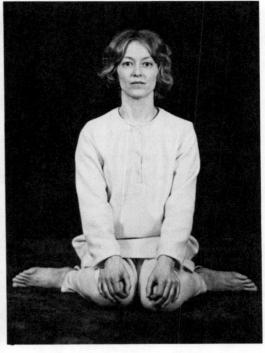

VIRASANA—WARRIOR POSTURE
Position 1

VIRASANA—WARRIOR POSTURE
Position 2

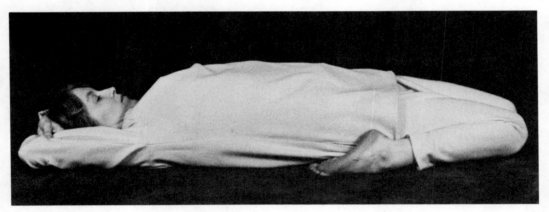

SUPTA VIRASANA—RECLINING WARRIOR POSTURE

57

MANDUKĀSANA/Frog

Kneel with the feet and shins on the floor. Bring the knees as far apart as possible. Place the feet in such a way that the heels are on the outside of the buttocks and the large toes touch behind the body. The buttocks should be firmly on the floor and not resting on the heels.

Place the palms on the knees; keep the spine erect. Hold for 15 seconds and slowly increase to one minute.

Benefits
- The frog and warrior's postures are very beneficial for increasing the flexibility of the ankles, knees, and hips.

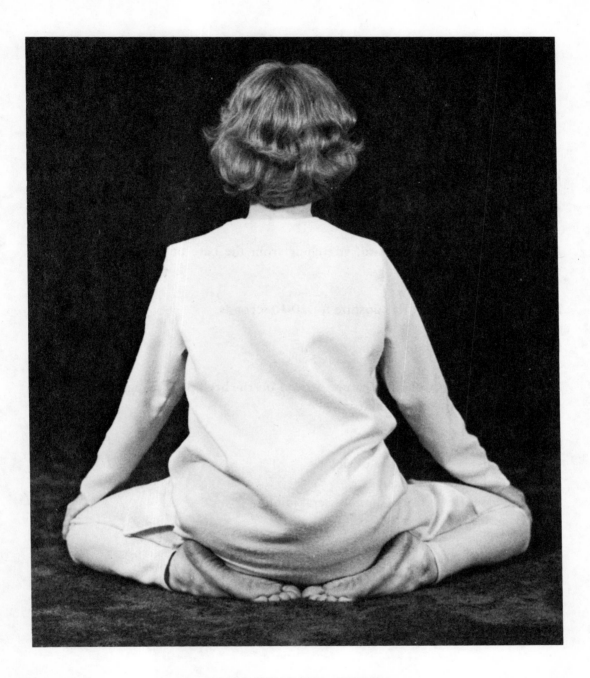

MANDUKASANA—FROG

YOGA MUDRĀ/Symbol of Yoga

Sit in *padmasana* (lotus posture).

Bring both arms behind the body and grasp the right wrist with the left hand.

Exhaling, slowly bend forward, stretching from the base of the spine. Rest the forehead on the floor.

Breathe evenly; relax in this posture for 20-30 seconds.

Inhaling, slowly return to a sitting position.

NOTE: The benefits of this posture depend on the heels pressing against the abdomen at the inside of the hip joints.

Benefits
- Stimulates the digestive organs
- Stretches the lower spine
- Increases flexibility of lumbo-sacral joints
- Beneficial for constipation

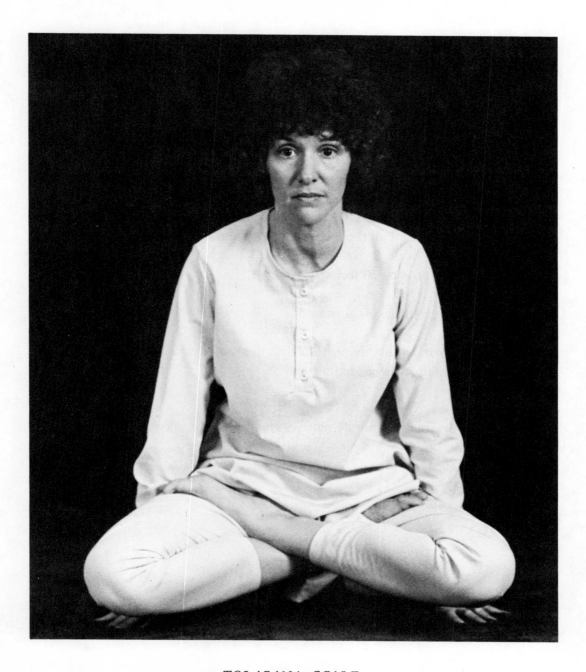

TOLASANA—SCALE

63

Preparation for
YOGANIDRĀ/Yogic Sleep

Sit with the head, neck, and trunk straight, legs extended in front of the body.

Bend the left leg; grasp the ankle with the left palm and the toes and ball of the foot with the right hand. Pull the foot to the forehead.

Breathe evenly; hold for 10-20 seconds.

Relax the leg. Repeat on the opposite side.

NOTE: It is important in this posture that the spine remains straight. The head should not be lowered to meet the foot.

Benefits
- Increases flexibility of all the muscles and joints of the legs and feet

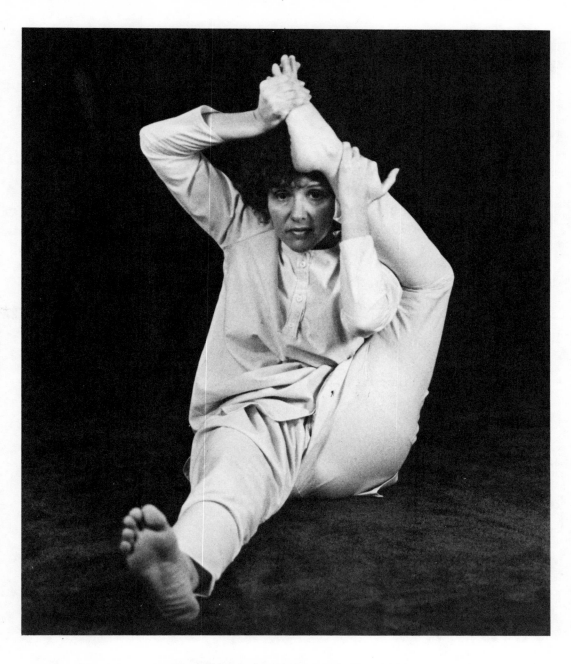

PREPARATION FOR *YOGANIDRA*

PADĀNDGUSHTĀSANA
Tiptoe Posture

Preparation

Squat, resting the weight of the body on the toes.
Place the hands at the hips and concentrate on a fixed point at eye level in front of the body. Hold for 30-60 seconds.

Posture

In the same position described above, place the left foot on the right thigh. Balance on the right toes for 2-5 seconds. Bring the hands to the chest in prayer position.

Repeat on the opposite side.

Gradually increase the time in this posture to 15 seconds.

Benefits
- Develops poise, concentration, and balance
- Strengthens the muscles of the legs, especially around the ankles
- Increases flexibility of the ankles and knees

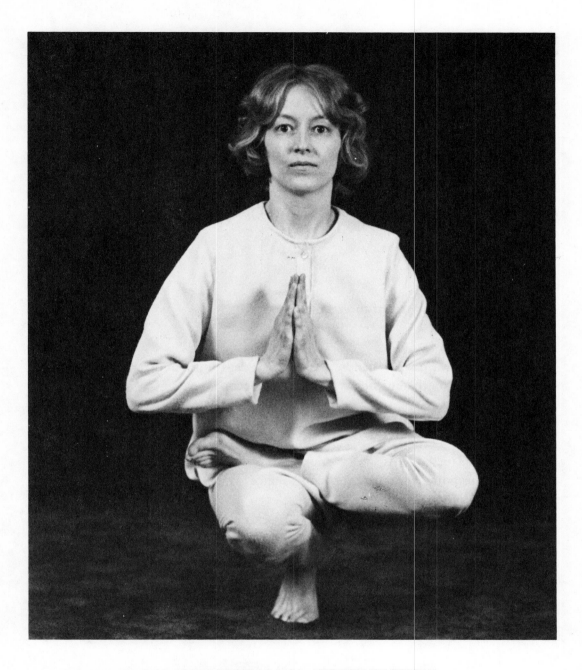

PADANDGUSHTASANA—TIPTOE POSTURE

67

SANTULĀNGĀSANA/Balance Posture

Preparation

Sit with the knees bent, soles of the feet together. Grasp the right heel with the right hand. Extend the leg upward and outward until both the arm and leg are straight. Hold for 3-5 seconds.

Repeat with the opposite leg.

Repeat on each side a total of three times.

Posture

Grasp both heels with the hands. Extend the legs until both arms and legs are straight. Balance on the buttocks. Hold for 3-5 seconds.

Repeat a total of three times.

Benefits
- Develops poise, concentration, and balance
- Stretches the calf and hamstring muscles
- Strengthens the abdominal and lower back muscles

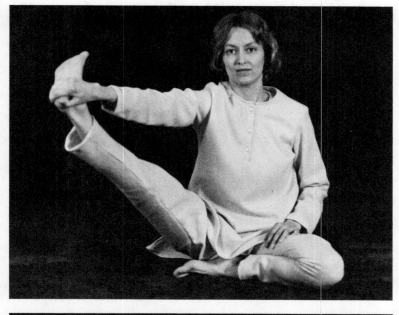

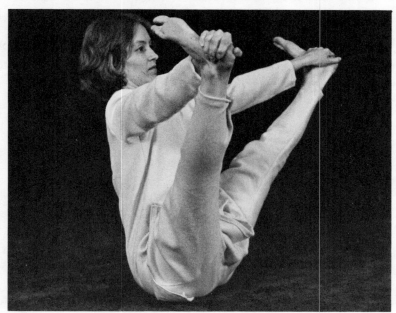

SANTULANGASANA—BALANCE POSTURE

69

URDHVĀSANA/Back Bending Posture

Stand firmly with the head, neck, and trunk in a straight line, feet together.

Inhaling, stretch the arms overhead until they are next to the ears. Keeping the legs straight, and the head between the arms, arch the spine and bend back as far as possible without straining.

Breathe evenly; hold for 10-15 seconds.

Exhaling, lower the arms. Relax.

Benefits
- This backbending posture uses gravity to help you go into the posture. It allows you to concentrate particularly on relaxation and gently moving to the limit of the spine's flexibility.

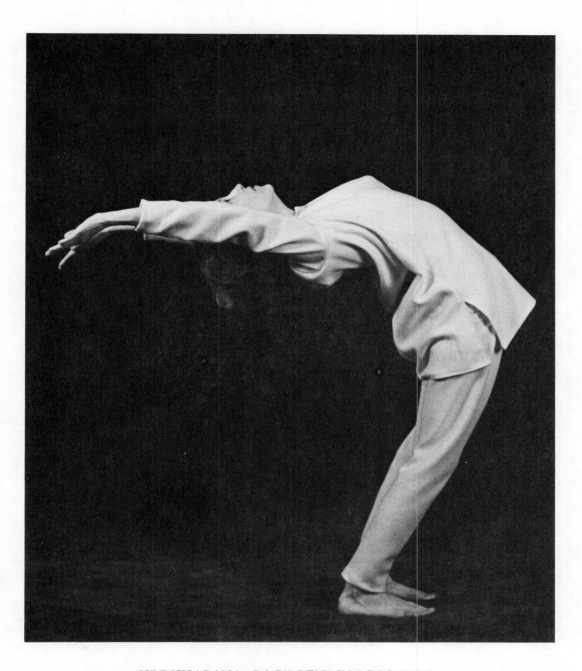

URDHVASANA—BACK BENDING POSTURE

71

Preparation for
USTRĀSANA/Camel

Kneel with the legs together.

With the fingers pointing down, place the heels of the hands on either side of the spine just above the buttocks.

Exhaling, gently bend back from the waist allowing the head to hang loosely.

Breathe evenly; hold for 10 seconds.

Inhaling, slowly raise.

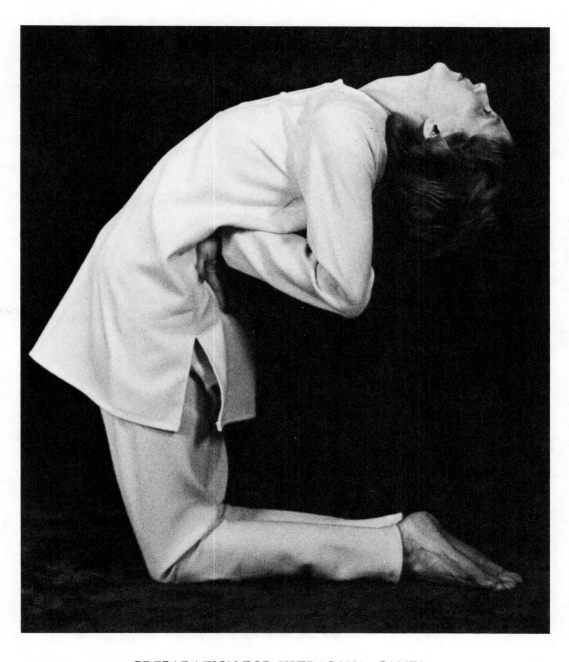

PREPARATION FOR *USTRASANA*—CAMEL

73

USTRĀSANA/Camel

Kneel with the legs together.

Exhaling, slowly bend back from the waist and place the palms on the soles of the feet.

Breathe evenly; hold for 10-20 seconds.

Follow the camel posture with *balasana* (child's posture, page 122 of the *Hatha Yoga Manual I*).

NOTE: This posture can also be done by grasping the ankles with the hands.

Benefits
- Develops flexibility of the spine
- Especially good for people with rounded shoulders
- The chest is expanded, promoting deep inhalation, giving good ventilation to the top of the lungs, and increasing their capacity.

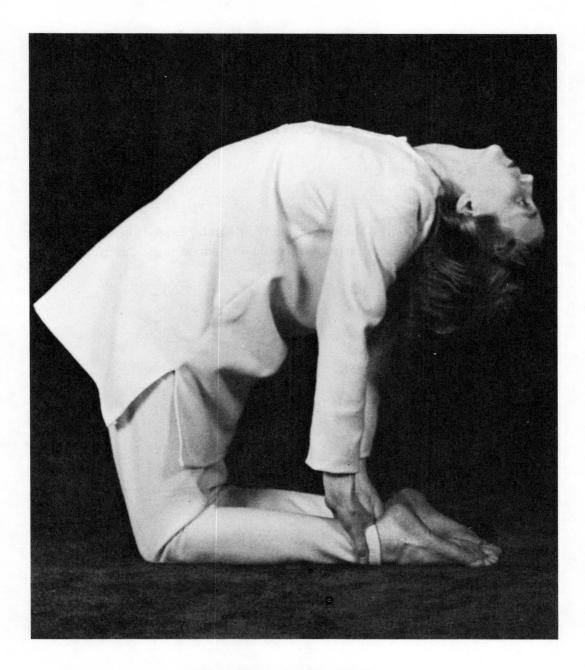

USTRASANA—CAMEL POSTURE

Preparation for
POORNA SUPTA VAJRĀSANA
Full Kneeling Posture

Preparatory Exercise 1
Kneel on the floor.

Leaning back, grasp the right ankle with the right hand. Extend the left arm next to the ear. Stretch back and attempt to hold the left arm parallel to the floor. Hold for 3-5 seconds.

Repeat on the opposite side.

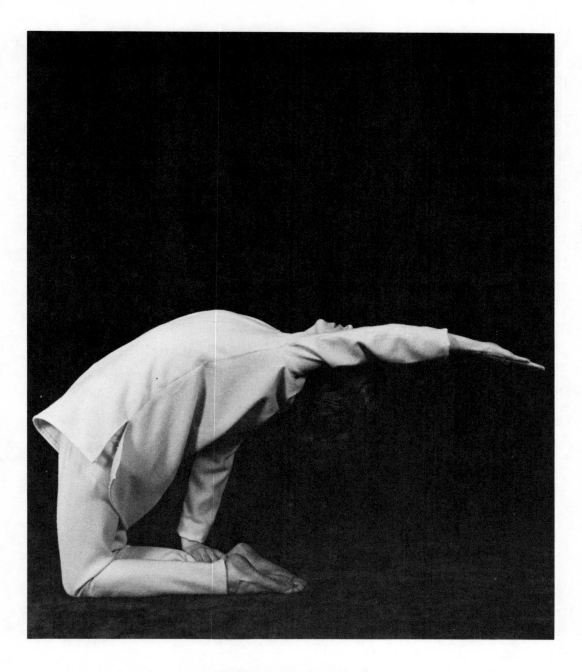

PREPARATION FOR
POORNA SUPTA VAJRASANA—FULL KNEELING POSTURE
Exercise 1

Preparatory Exercise 2
Kneel on the floor.

Stretch both arms above the head. Keeping the arms next to the ears, slowly bend back until the hands are resting on the floor. Hold for 3-5 seconds.

Initially one may relax by lowering the body until the back is on the floor. As strength and flexibility increase, practice raising the body and returning to a kneeling position. Slowly try to bring the hands closer and closer to the feet. In the full kneeling posture, the hands rest on the feet.

Benefits
- Similar to *ustrasana*—camel posture
- Exercise 2 also strengthens the arms and wrists.

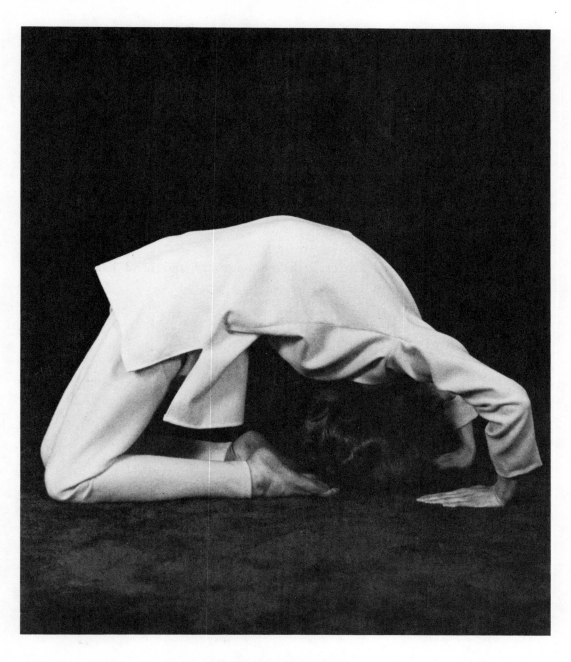

PREPARATION FOR
POORNA SUPTA VAJRASANA—FULL KNEELING POSTURE
Exercise 2

79

ARDHA-KAPOTĀSANA
Half Pigeon Posture

Sit in *vajrasana* (kneeling posture).

Place the left heel at the perineum and extend the right leg straight back.
Place the hands on the waist.

Inhaling, expand the chest. Stretch the chin upward and bend back as far as possible.

Breathe evenly; hold for 10-20 seconds.

Return to the kneeling posture.

Repeat on the opposite side.

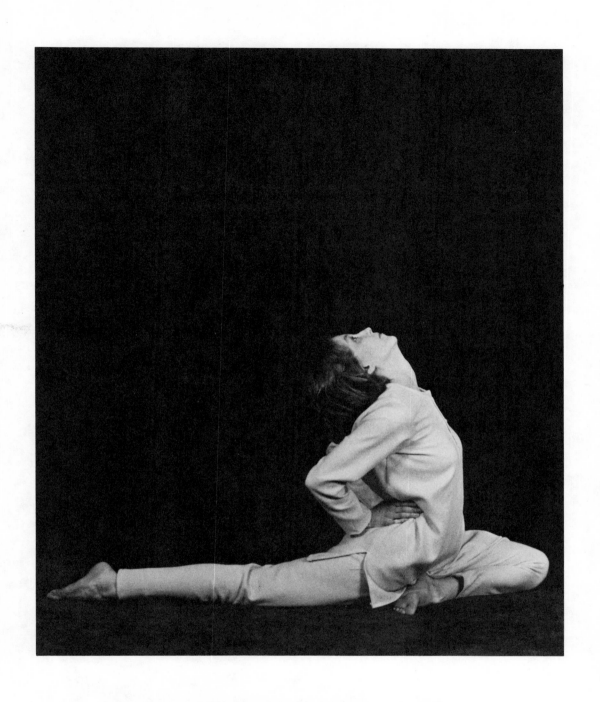

ARDHA-KAPOTASANA—HALF PIGEON POSTURE

Preparation for
KAPOTĀSANA/Pigeon Posture

A more advanced variation of *kapotasana* is to bend the leg which is extended, grasp the foot with the hands, and bring it to the head. The following is a preparatory exercise for this posture.

Bend the left knee and place the foot flat on the floor. Extend the right leg behind the body. Let the hands rest on the floor a few inches behind the left foot.

Inhaling, come up on the finger tips and bend back as far as possible. Now, bend the right leg and bring it to the head.

Breathe evenly; hold for 5-10 seconds.

Relax, and repeat on the opposite side.

Benefits
- Similar to *ustasana*—camel posture
- Stretches thigh muscles and pelvic ligaments

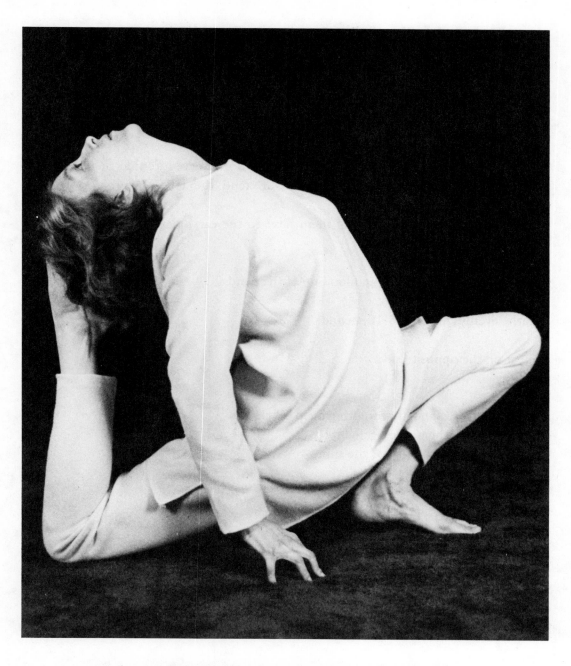

PREPARATION FOR KAPOTASANA—PIGEON POSTURE

83

BANARĀSANA/Monkey Posture

Bend the right knee with the foot flat on the floor. Make sure that the lower right leg remains perpendicular to the floor. Extend the left leg behind the body.

Inhaling, raise the arms and bring them next to the ears; place the hands in prayer position.

Exhaling, gently bend back and look up at the hands.

Breathe evenly; hold for 5-10 seconds.

Repeat on the opposite side.

Benefits
- Chest is expanded promoting deep inhalation
- Stretches the pelvic ligaments
- Develops flexibility of the spine

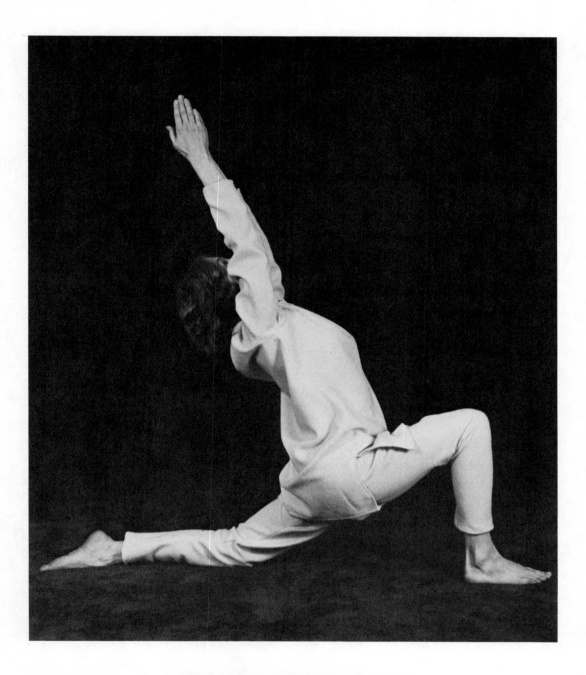

BANARASANA—MONKEY POSTURE

85

CHAKRĀSANA/Wheel

Lie on the back with the arms stretched over the head.

Bend the knees and bring the feet to the buttocks, shoulder width apart. Bend the arms and place the hands palms down, with the fingertips touching the shoulders.

Inhaling, progressively lift the buttocks, waist, and chest until the arms are straight. The head hangs between the arms.

Breathe evenly; hold for 10-20 seconds.

Exhaling, progressively lower the body first to the shoulders, then to the buttocks. Relax in the child's posture.

Variation
Repeat the posture as described above. Once in the posture, lift up onto the balls of the feet, hold for 5 seconds. Relax.

Benefits
- Stretches the whole spine
- Strengthens the arms and legs
- An excellent posture for people with rounded shoulders
- Increases the blood pressure and flow of blood to the brain

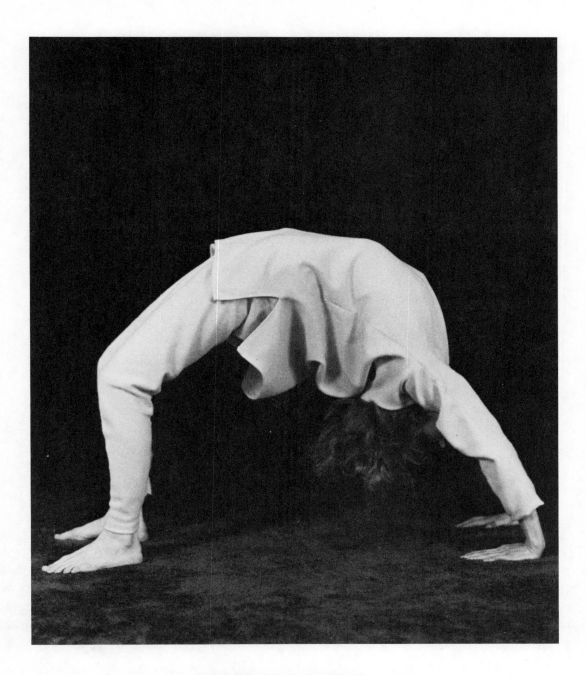

CHAKRASANA—WHEEL

87

Preparation for
Forward Bending Postures

Lie on the floor with the arms extended outward from the shoulders.

Raise the right leg. Keeping both legs straight, bring the right leg to the left hand. Hold for 5-10 seconds. Bring the leg back to center and slowly lower as in the leg lifts.

Repeat with the left leg.

Repeat on each side a total of three times.

Benefits
* Stretches hamstring and calf muscles

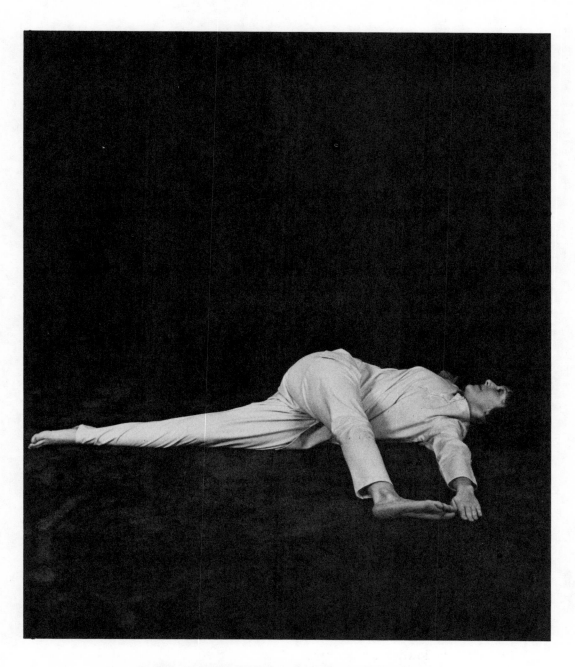

PREPARATION FOR FORWARD BENDING

89

BHADRĀSANA/Ankle~Knee Posture

First Position
Bending the knees, place the soles of the feet together; bring the heels as close to the body as possible. Interlace the fingers and place them around the toes. Draw the knees to the floor.

Exhaling, bend forward from the hips. Place the elbows on the floor and the fore-head on the feet.
Breathe evenly; hold for 10-20 seconds.
Inhaling, return to an upright position.

Second Position
Sit as described in the first position.

Inhaling, stretch the arms over the head.
Exhaling, bend forward stretching from the base of the spine. Bring the head to the floor and stretch the arms forward as far as possible.
Breathe evenly; hold for 10 seconds.

Inhaling, keeping the spine straight and the head between the arms, raise the body.

Lower the arms and return to a sitting position. Relax.

Benefits
- Increases flexibility of the hips and pelvis
- Stretches the inner thigh muscles
- Stretches the lower back and spine
- Strengthens abdominal muscles
- Increases flexibility of the knees and ankles
- Helps normalize menstrual flow

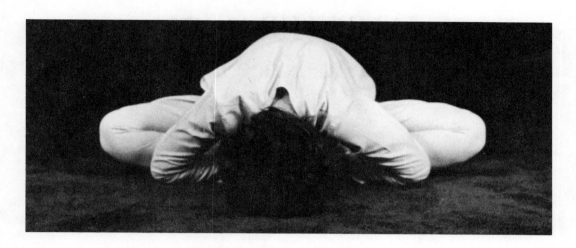

BHADRASANA—ANKLE-KNEE POSTURE
First Position

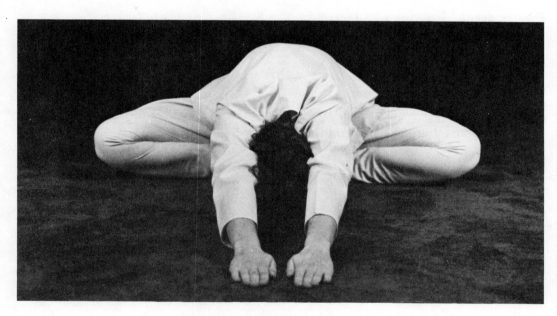

BHADRASANA—ANKLE-KNEE POSTURE
Second Position

91

JANUSHIRĀSANA
Head~to~Knee Posture

First Position

Sit with the legs extended. Bend the left leg and place heel snugly against the perineum.

Inhaling, raise both arms to the sides.

Exhaling, bend from the hips and place the right arm, palm up, against the inside of the right leg. As the body is lowered, bring the left arm next to the head and grasp the outside of the right foot, fingers extending to the instep.

Breathe evenly; hold for 10-20 seconds.

Repeat on the opposite side.

Second Position

Repeat the posture as described above, only place the right arm on the outside of the right leg and grasp the heel and toes with the hands.

Benefits
- Increases rotational flexibility of the spine
- Aids digestion
- Stretches the muscles along the side of the torso and the arms

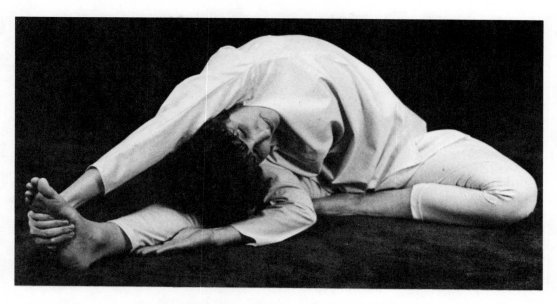

JANUSHIRASANA—HEAD-TO-KNEE POSTURE
First Position

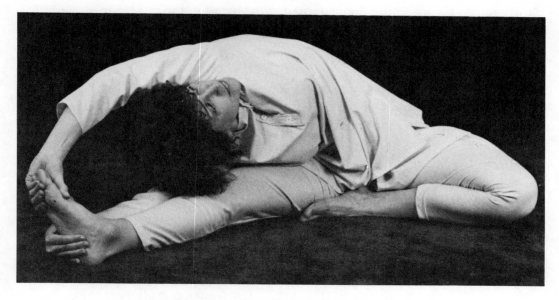

JANUSHIRASANA—HEAD-TO-KNEE POSTURE
Second Position

93

Third Position

Sit with the head, neck, and trunk straight; extend the legs keeping both knees flat on the floor.

Beginning at the thigh, "walk" the hands up the right leg until both hands grasp the foot and the leg is pulled close to the face. Keep the knees straight.

Breathe evenly; hold for 20 seconds.

Slowly return the leg to the floor alternating the hands in the same manner described above.

Repeat on the opposite side.

NOTE: The most benefit is received from this posture if the leg is pulled to the face rather than the head lowered to the leg.

Benefits
- Increases flexibility of the hamstrings and calf muscles
- Strengthens abdominal and lower back muscles.

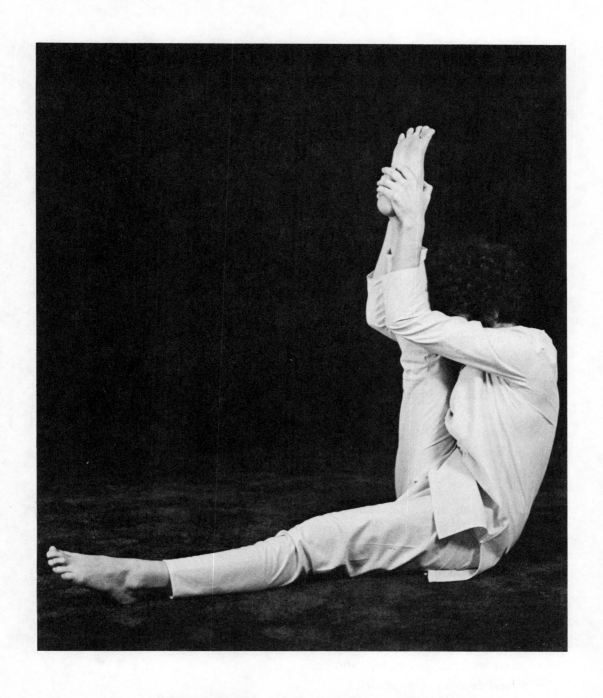

JANUSHIRASANA—HEAD-TO-KNEE POSTURE
Third Position

95

UPAVISTHA KONĀSANA
Spread Leg Stretches

First Position

Sit with the head, neck, and trunk straight. Spread the legs as far apart as possible; rest the hands on the knees.

Inhaling, raise the arms out to the sides to shoulder level. Exhaling, bend forward from the hips until the chin rests on the floor. Grasp the inner arch of the foot with the fingers.
Breathe evenly; hold for 20 seconds.
Inhaling, and keeping the spine straight, slowly return to a sitting position.

NOTE: In all spread-leg postures it is important to stretch from the base of the spine rather than just bending forward from the waist.

Second Position

Sit in the position described above. Raise the arms out to the sides to shoulder level.

Inhaling, draw the arms behind the body and entwine the fingers.
Exhaling, bend forward and stretch from the base of the spine until the forehead rests on the floor.
Breathe evenly; hold for 20 seconds.

Keeping the spine straight, return to a sitting position.

Benefits
- Increases flexibility of hips and pelvis
- Stretches inner thigh muscles
- Stretches lower back and spine
- Strengthens abdominal muscles

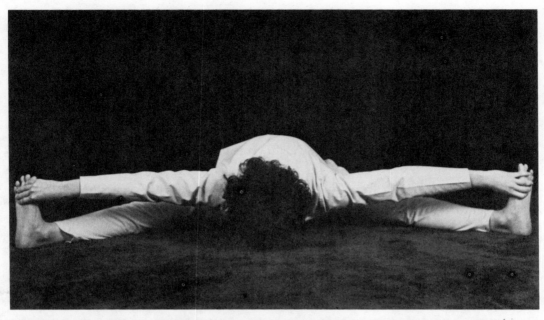

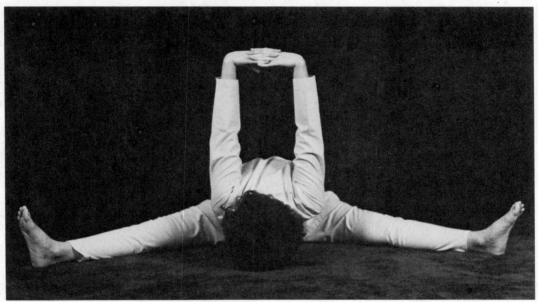

UPAVISTHA KONASANA—SPREAD LEG STRETCHES

97

KURMĀSANA/Tortoise

Sit with the head, neck, and trunk straight; spread the legs as far apart as possible.

Exhaling, and stretching forward from the base of the spine, insert the left arm, palm down, beneath the left leg. Repeat with the right. Place the chin on the floor and pull the chest as close to the floor as possible.

Breathe evenly; hold for 10 seconds.

Inhaling, return to a sitting position.

Benefits
  • Same as *upavistha konasana*

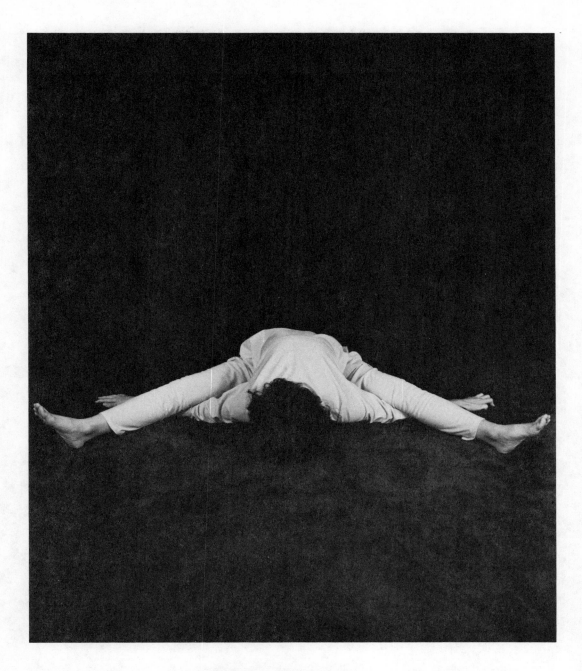

KURMASANA—TORTOISE

99

ĀKARṆA DHANURĀSANA
Archer Posture

First Position

Sit with the head, neck, and trunk straight; extend the legs straight in front of the body.

Exhaling, reach forward with both arms and grasp the big toes with the index fingers.

Inhaling, gently pull the right toe to the right ear. Hold firmly onto the left toe and keep the leg flat on the floor.

Breathe evenly; hold for 20 seconds.

Repeat on the opposite side.

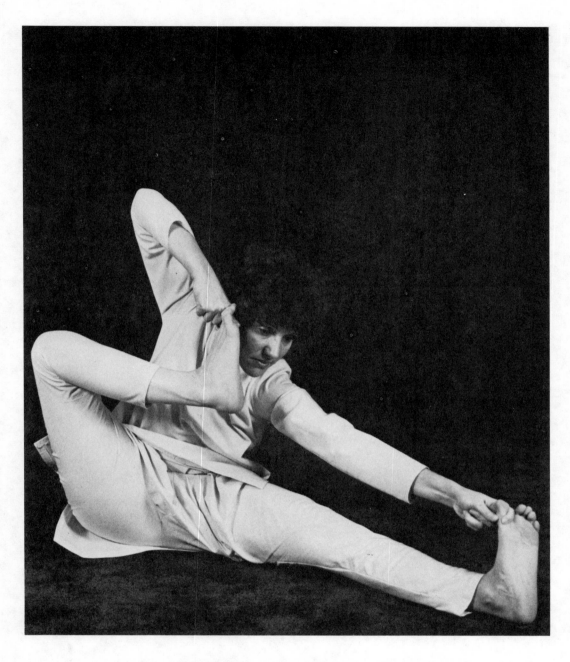

AKARNA DHANURASANA—ARCHER POSTURE
First Position

Second Position

Repeat the first position with this variation: grasp the right big toe with the left index finger. Reach under the left arm and grasp the left big toe with the right index finger.

Inhaling, gently pull the left toe to the right ear.

Breathe evenly; hold for 20 seconds.

Repeat on the opposite side.

Benefits
- Increases flexibility in all the muscles of the legs
- Increases flexibility of the ankle, knee, and hip joints

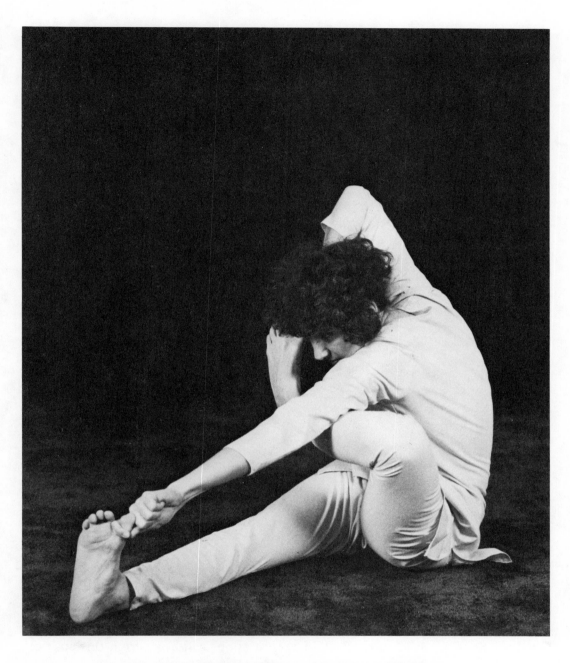

AKARNA DHANURASANA—ARCHER POSTURE
Second Position

103

HALĀSANA/Plow

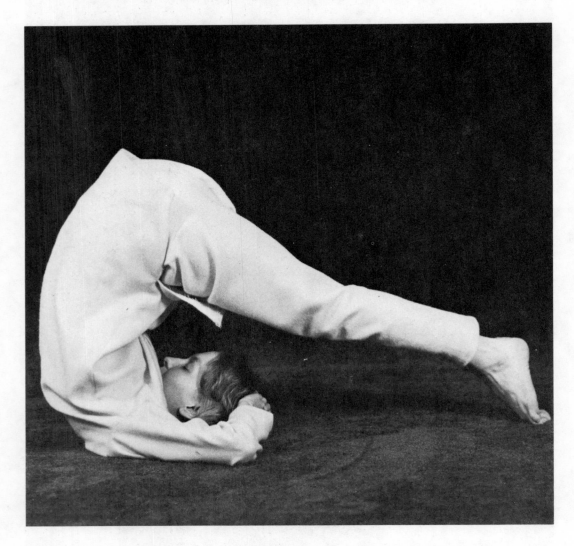

Assume the plow posture as described in *Hatha Yoga Manual I*, p 102. Breathe evenly; hold for two minutes. Each of the variations will begin from this position.

Variation 1
Interlace the fingers and place them above the head. Point the toes away from the head. Breathe evenly; hold for 30 seconds.

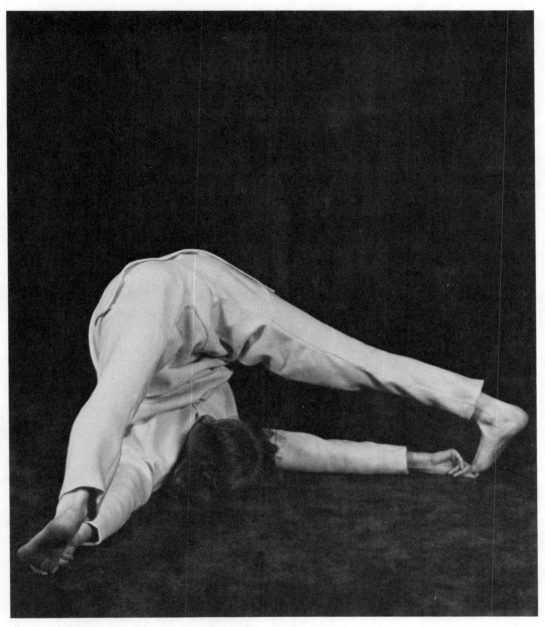

HALASANA—PLOW
Variation 2

Spread the legs to form a "V" and grasp the large toes with the index fingers. Breathe evenly; hold for 30 seconds.

105

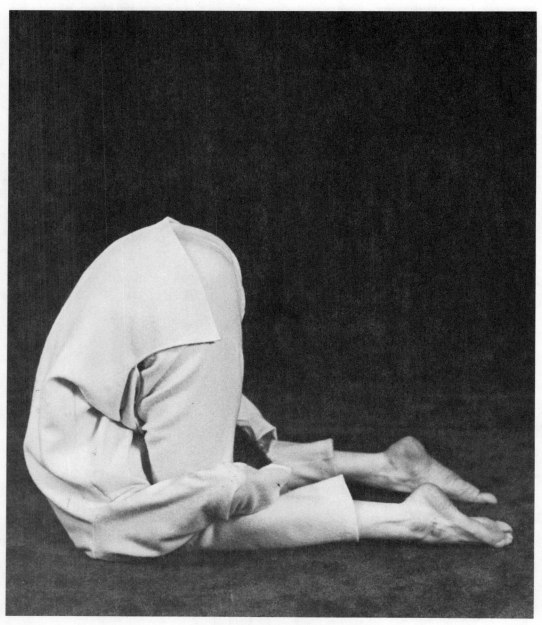

HALASANA—PLOW
Variation 3

Bend the knees and place them on the floor beside the ears. Place the arms over the knees and cover the ears with the hands. Breathe evenly; hold for 30 seconds.

106

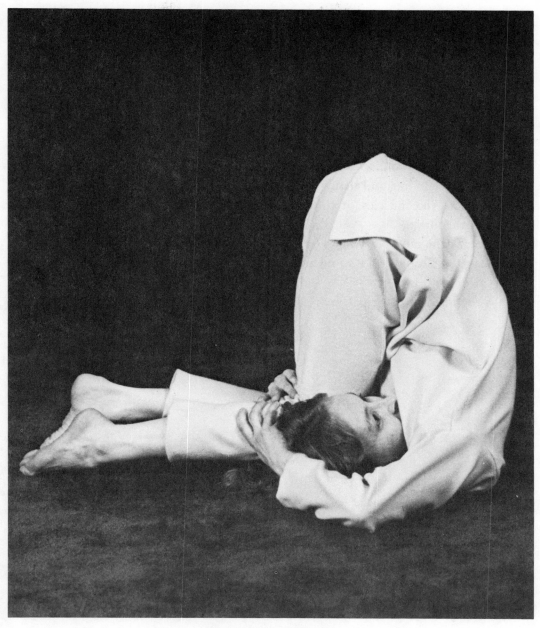

HALASANA—PLOW
Variation 4

Bend both knees and place them beside the right ear. Breathe evenly; hold for 30 seconds. Repeat on the left side.

Variation 5

Raise the right leg until it is perpendicular to the floor. Keep both legs straight. Breathe evenly; hold for 30 seconds.

Repeat with the opposite leg.

Slowly come out of the plow posture. Relax completely.

Benefits
- Lengthens the muscles of the back of the thighs and prepares the body for forward bending and sitting postures.
- Relaxes the muscles of the back and gently stretches the ligaments of the spinal column
- One of the most reviving and rejuvenating of all postures
- Massages, tones, and stimulates all internal organs, especially the intestines, spleen, and liver
- Beneficial for constipation

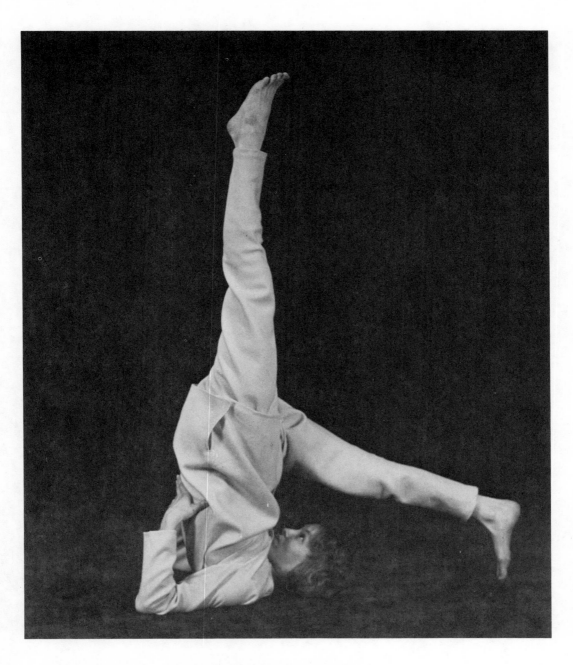

HALASANA—PLOW
Variation 5

SARVANGĀSANA/Shoulderstand

Variation 1

Lie on the back, place the arms palms down along the sides of the body with the legs together.

Inhaling, slowly raise both legs until they are perpendicular to the floor. Then, lift the hips, the lower, middle, and upper spine until only the shoulders rest on the floor. Keep the legs straight and together.

Breathe evenly; hold for two minutes.

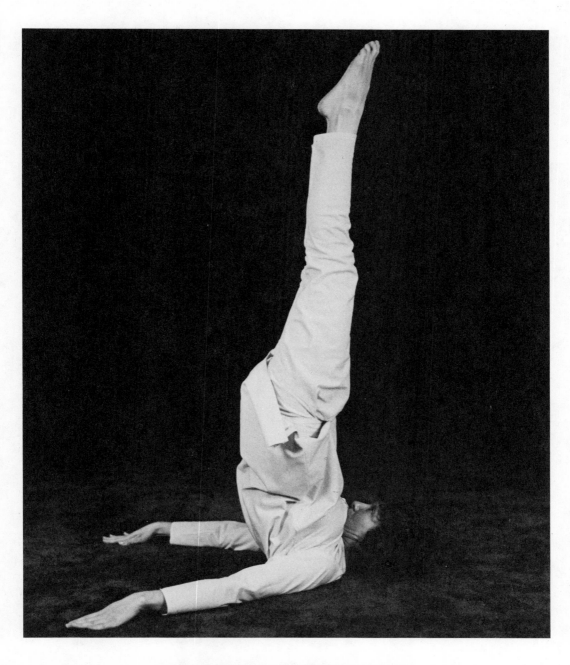

SARVANGASANA—SHOULDERSTAND
Variation 1

111

Variation 2
Spread the legs to form a "V".

Breathe evenly; hold for 20 seconds.

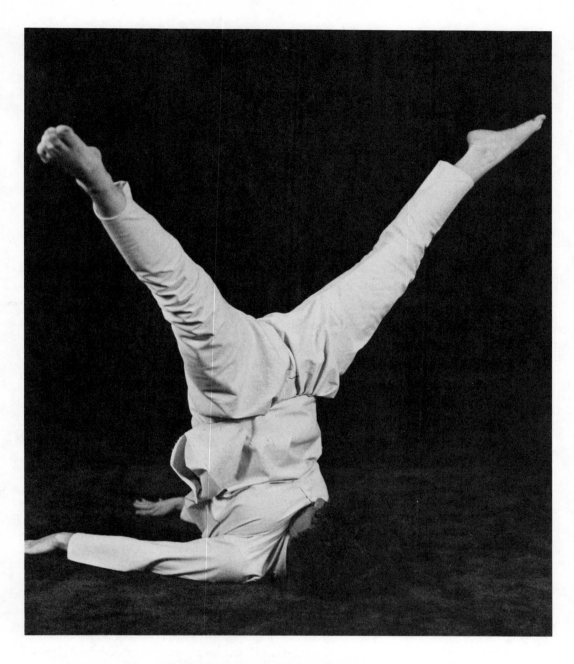

SARVANGASANA−SHOULDERSTAND
Variation 2

Variation 3

Bend the knees and place the soles of the feet together. Twist the body to the right. Hold for 10 seconds.

Repeat, twisting in the opposite direction.

Return to *sarvangasana* as described in variation 1.

Exhaling, slowly lower the hips and return the legs to a perpendicular position. Continue exhaling and lower the legs to the floor.

Benefits
- As implied in the literal translation of *sarvangasana*, "all members posture," this posture benefits all parts of the body, the shoulders, arms, legs, head, neck, back, and internal organs
- Strengthens arms, chest, and shoulders
- Slims legs and hips
- Strengthens back and abdominal muscles
- Places gentle traction on the cervical vertebrae, keeping this important area healthy and flexible
- Venous drainage of the legs occurs quickly and completely, especially benefitting those with varicose veins
- As in the inverted action posture, diaphragmatic breathing is easily observed and learned
- Causes higher blood pressure and simple mechanical pressure in the neck which are said to rejuvenate the thyroid and parathyroid glands, making them function optimally. These important glands regulate body weight and metabolism by natural mechanisms
- Reduces the occurrence of acute and chronic throat ailments
- Increases blood supply to all the important structures of the neck
- Considered by hatha yoga literature to be the "Queen of Asanas" and a panacea for internal organ ailments, especially those of old age. The shoulderstand combats indigestion, constipation, degeneration of endocrine glands, problems occurring in the liver, the gall bladder, the kidney, the pancreas, the spleen, and the digestive system

114

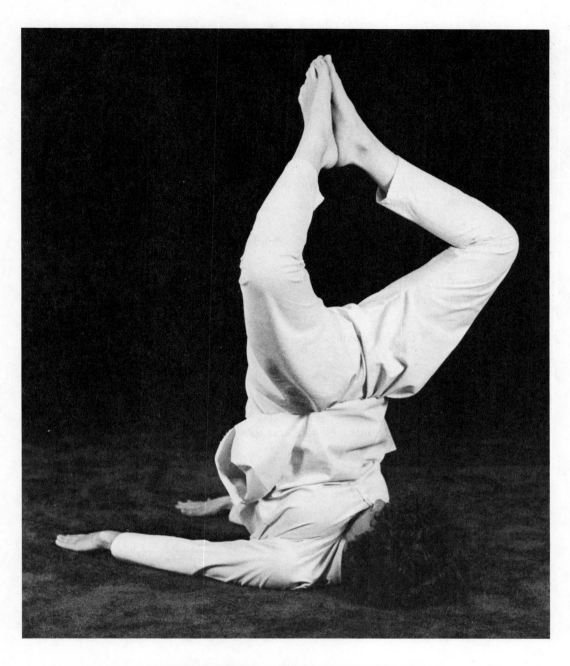

SARVANGASANA—SHOULDERSTAND
Variation 3

115

SETU/Bridge

Variation 1

Assume the unsupported shoulderstand posture. Place the hands on either side of the spine just above the waist.

Place the sole of the right foot on top of the left knee.

Exhaling, lower the left foot to the floor. Place the right foot on the floor beside the left; keep the legs together.

Breathe evenly; hold for 20 seconds.

NOTE: The legs can also be lowered without placing the foot on the knee.

Variation 2

Grasp the ankles with the hands. Be sure not to allow the back to sag.

Breathe evenly; hold for 10-15 seconds.

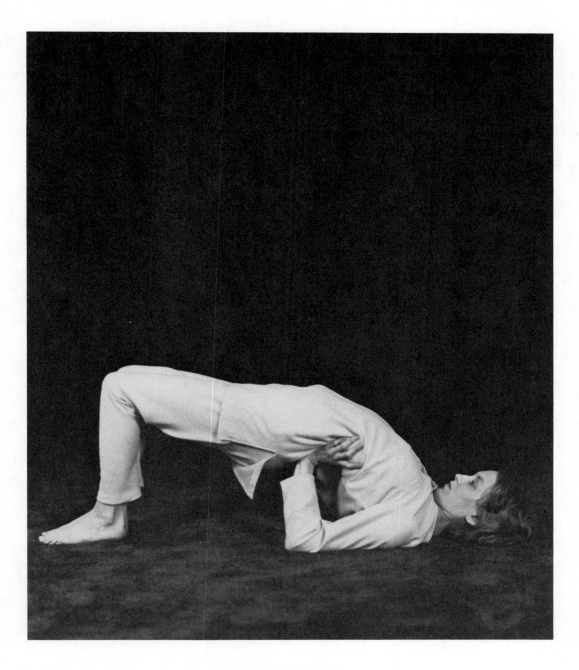

SETU–BRIDGE

117

Variation 3
Assume the bridge posture as in variation 1.

Exhaling, raise the right leg.

Breathe evenly; hold for 5-10 seconds.

Inhaling, slowly lower the leg.

Repeat with the opposite leg.

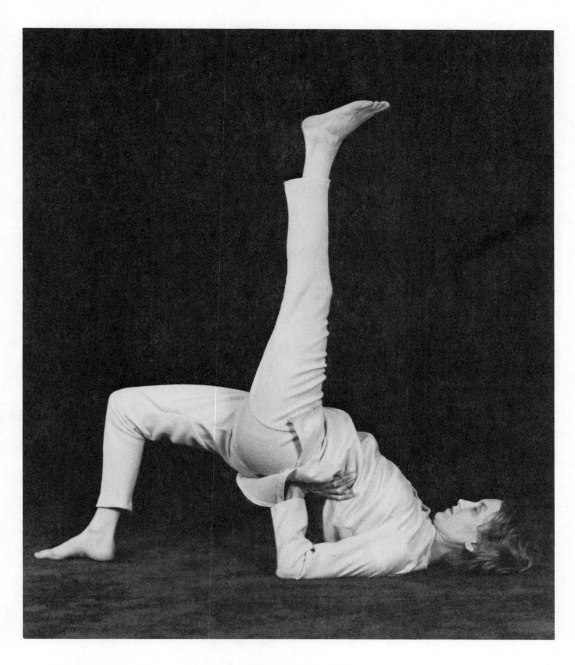

SETU−BRIDGE
Variation 3

119

Variation 4
Assume the bridge posture as described in variation 1.

Exhaling, stretch out both legs. Keep the legs together and the feet flat on the floor.

Breathe evenly; hold for 10 seconds.

Raise the legs and return to the shoulderstand posture.

Exhaling, slowly lower the hips and return the legs to a perpendicular position. Continue exhaling and lower the legs to the floor.

Follow the plow, shoulderstand, and bridge postures with the fish posture.

Benefits
Increases flexibility and circulation to the lower back.

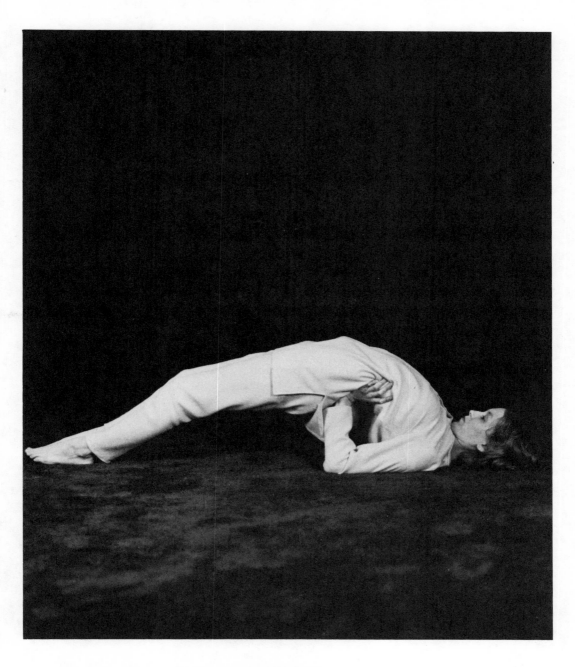

SETU−BRIDGE
Variation 4

121

ARDHA-MATSYĀSANA/Half Fish

Sit in a kneeling position with the head, neck, and trunk straight.

Exhaling, lean back and place the elbows on the floor behind the body. Inhaling, arch the back, expand the chest, and place the crown of the head on the floor.

Breathe evenly; hold the posture for the length of time it takes to relieve any tension in the neck and shoulders from the inverted postures. The amount of time the posture is held will vary according to the amount of time the student spent in the plow, shoulderstand, and bridge postures.

Raise the body and return to a kneeling position.

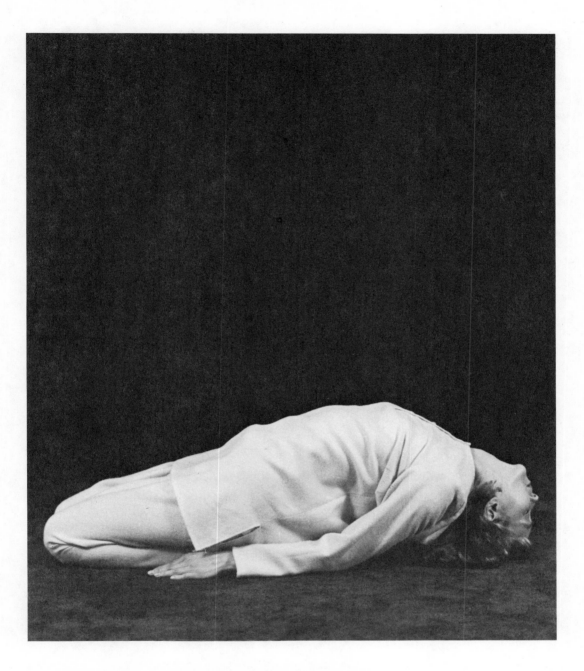

ARDHA-MATSYASANA—FISH

123

MATSYĀSANA/Fish

Sit in *padmasana*.

Exhaling, lean back and place the elbows on the floor.

Inhaling, arch the back, expand the chest, and place the crown of the head on the floor.

Take hold of the big toes with the index fingers and the thumbs. Keep the elbows on the floor.

Breathe evenly; hold for the length of time it takes to relieve any tension in the neck and shoulders.

Release the legs and relax the body completely.

Benefits
- Provides a stretch to the cervical vertebrae which complements that of the shoulderstand. It amplifies the effects of the shoulderstand and eliminates the slight stiffness in the neck and back which results from doing the shoulderstand alone
- The chest is thrown out, promoting deep inhalation, giving good ventilation to the top of the lungs, and increasing their capacity
- In *padmasana*: increases flexibility of hips, knees, and ankles

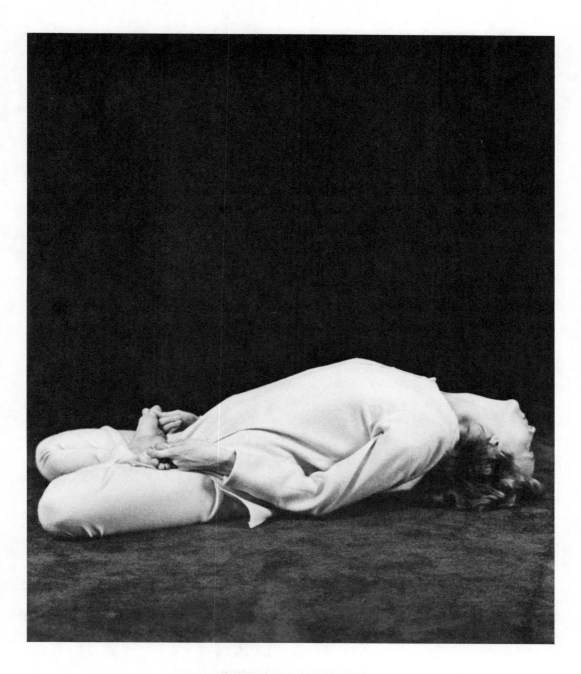

MATSYASANA—FISH

125

MATSYENDRĀSANA/Spinal Twist

Variation 1
Sit with the head, neck and trunk straight. Extend the legs in front of the body. Bend the left leg and place the left heel at the perineum. Bend the right leg and place the right foot on the floor outside the left knee. The toes of the right foot should extend slightly in front of the left knee.

Inhaling, raise the arms to shoulder level.
Exhaling, twist the body enough to the right to pass over the right knee and grasp the right foot with the left hand. Continue the twist, wrapping the right arm behind the body to grasp the waist.

Gaze over the right shoulder with the chin parallel to the floor. Breathe evenly; hold for 30 seconds.

Variation 2
Repeat the posture with this variation:
Twist the body enough to the right to pass over the right knee. Bend the left elbow; reach under the right knee and clasp the hands behind the back.

Breathe evenly; hold for 30 seconds.
Relax the arms and legs.

Benefits
- Provides a twist to the spinal column, stretching and lengthening the muscles and ligaments and keeping the spine elastic and healthy
- Alternately compresses each half of the abdominal region, squeezing those internal organs and promoting better circulation through them
- Combats constipation, reduces fat and improves digestion
  Massages the kidneys

126

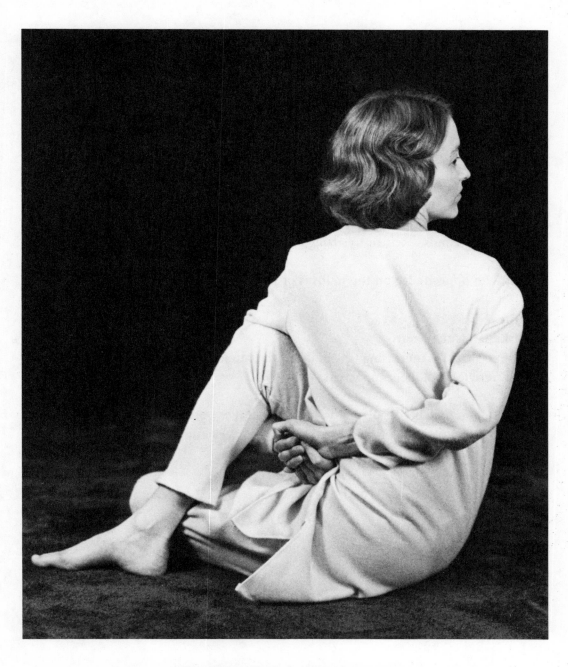

MATSYENDRASANA—SPINAL TWIST
Variation 2

127

LUPTA PADMĀSANA/Hidden Lotus

Sit in the lotus posture.

Raise up on the knees and bring the body forward until the front of the legs, chest, and chin are on the floor.   Place the hands behind the back in the prayer position.* Hold for 10 seconds. Return to sitting posture.

Repeat with opposite leg on top in lotus posture.

Benefits
- Expands the chest
- Excellent for increasing flexibility of the hip joints
- Stretches shoulders and wrists

*If it is uncomfortable to place the hands in prayer position, fold the arms in front of the body and place the forehead on the forearms as in the crocodile posture.

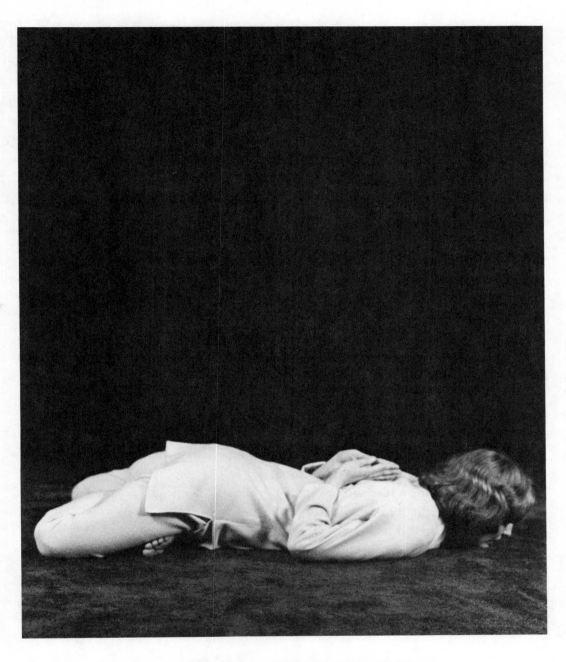

LUPTA PADMASANA—HIDDEN LOTUS

129

SIMHĀSANA PADMĀSANA
Lion in Lotus Posture

Sit in *padmasana* with both hands by the sides.

Lift the buttocks from the floor and walk the hands forward until they are two feet in front of the knees.

*Exhaling, open the mouth as wide as possible and thrust the tongue out and down, trying to touch the chin.

Gaze at a point between the eyebrows.

Inhaling, close the mouth and relax the face. Take one complete breath. Repeat from * two more times. Relax the body.

Benefits
- Makes the voice soft and melodious
- Releases tension in neck and throat area, especially beneficial for people who have a feeling of a lump in their throat
- Aids in relieving a sore throat
- Increases flexibility of hip joints
- Is said to cure bad breath

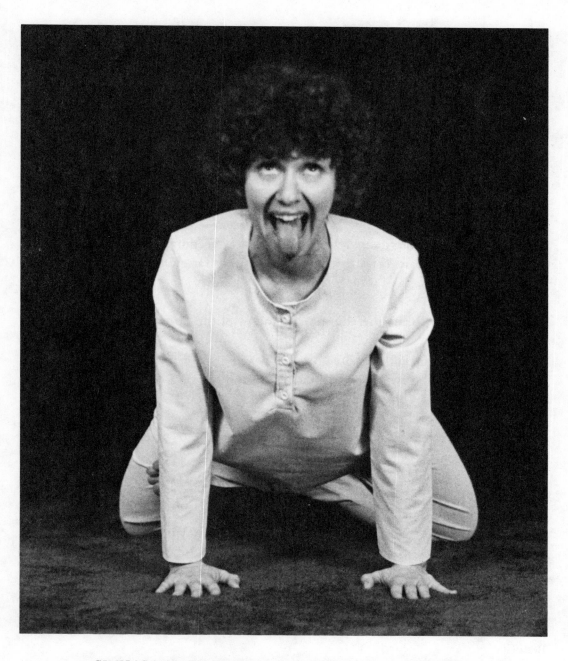

SIMHASANA PADMASANA—LION IN LOTUS POSTURE

131

AGNISARA

Agnisara is similar to *uddiyana bandha* (abdominal Lift) as described in *Hatha Yoga Manual I* on page 134. In *agnisara*, however, the abdominal muscles are contracted and released a number of times without inhaling.

Stand with the feet approximately two feet apart. Keeping the spine straight, bend the knees slightly; lean forward from the waist only far enough to place the palms just above the knees.

Exhale completely, place the chin on the hollow of the throat, and hold the breath.

Without inhaling, suck the abdominal muscles in and up, pulling the navel toward the spine. This motion pulls the diaphragm up and creates a cavity on the front side of the abdomen under the rib cage.

Release and then contract the abdominal muscles 6-10 times without inhaling. Slowly inhale and relax.

Repeat three times.

As in *uddiyana bandha* it is important to use force only when pulling the abdominal muscles in, never force the muscles outward. Do not practice this exercise if you have high blood pressure, hiatal hernia, ulcers, or heart disorders. Women should not practice it during menstruation or pregnancy. It has been found that this exercise may be irritating to women with IUD's.

Benefits
  • Promotes health in all the internal organs
  • Stimulates digestion

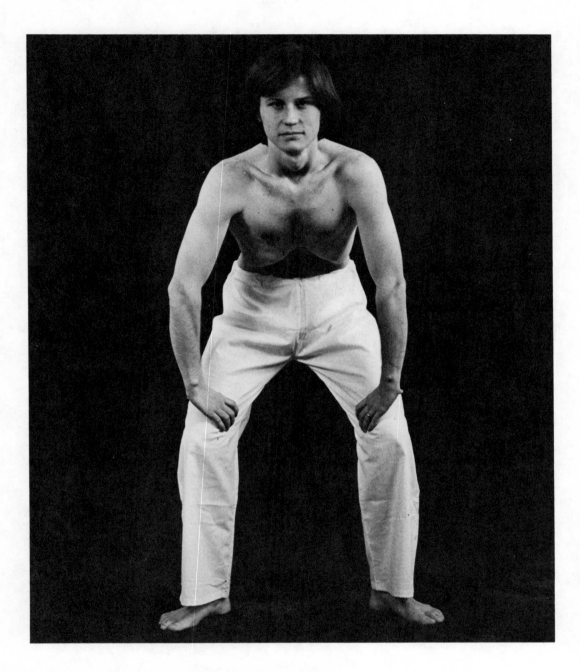

AGNISARA

133

BHUJAPĪDĀSANA/Crow

Stand with the legs shoulder width apart.

Bend the knees and place the palms on the floor six inches apart. Spread the fingers for balance.

Exhaling, lean forward and place the upper thighs on the upper arms. Lift the feet from the floor balancing the weight of the body on the hands. Point the toes and draw them together until they touch.

Breathe evenly; hold for 5-10 seconds.

Lower the feet and return to a standing position.

Benefits
- Strengthens the arms, shoulders, and wrists
- Strengthens abdominal muscles

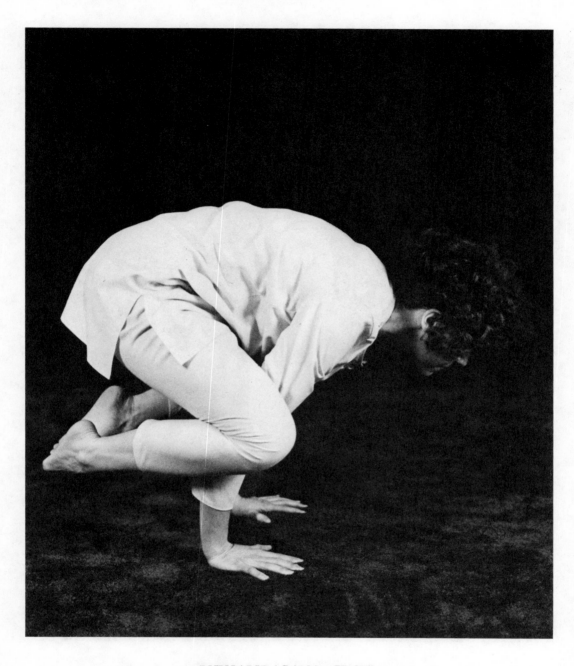

BHUJAPIDASANA—CROW

135

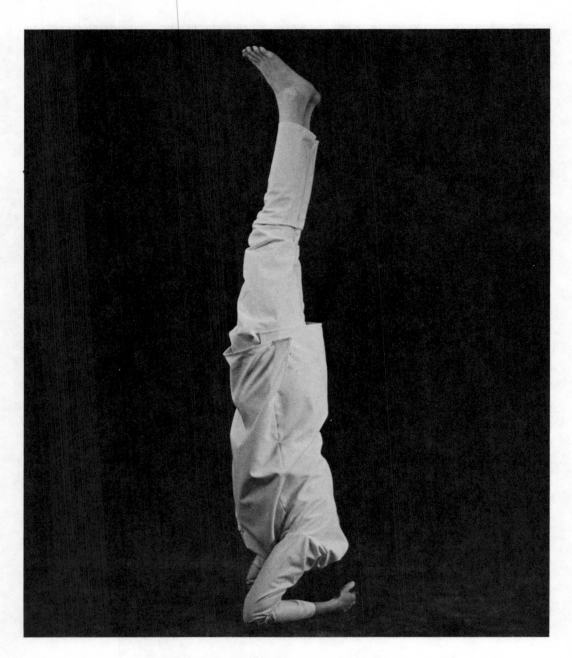

SHIRSHĀSANA / Headstand

Follow the directions for the headstand posture in *Hatha Yoga Manual I.*

136

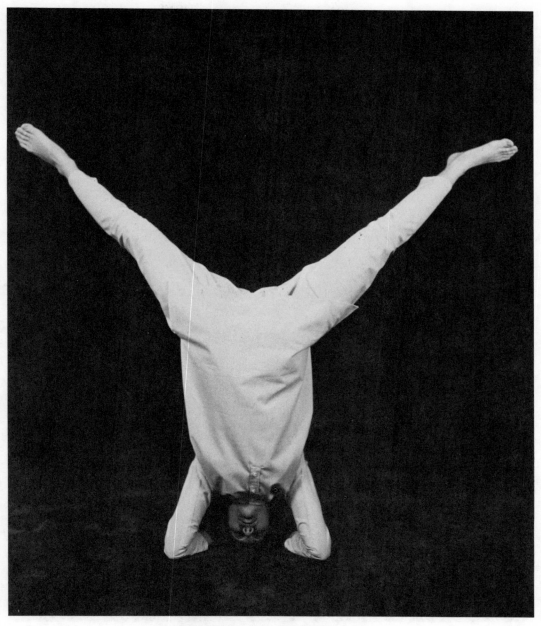

SHIRSHASANA—HEADSTAND
Variation 1

Assume the headstand posture. Spread the legs to form a "V". Rotate the ankles. Relax the feet. Breathe evenly; hold for 30 seconds. Bring the legs together.

137

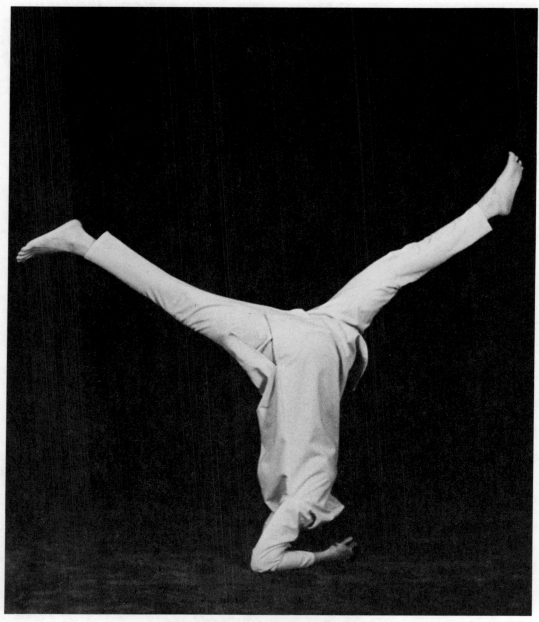

SHIRSHASANA—HEADSTAND
Variation 2

Spread the legs as in the splits. Breathe evenly; hold for 5 seconds. Raise the legs and repeat with the opposite leg coming forward. Bring the legs together.

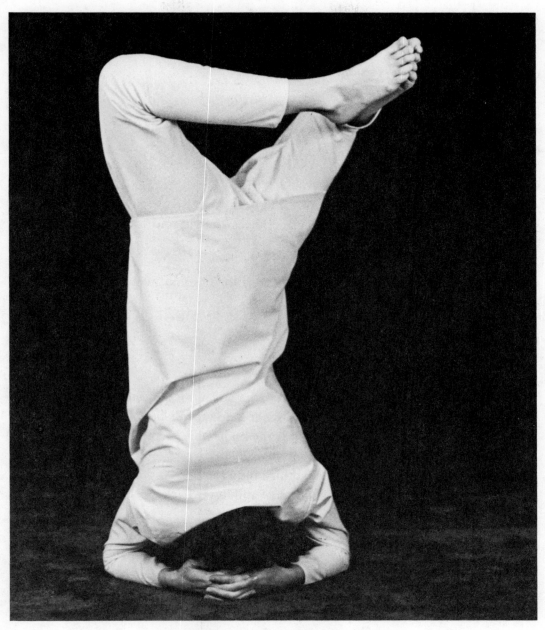

SHIRSHASANA—HEADSTAND
Variation 3

Bend the knees and bring the soles of the feet together. Twist the lower torso to the right until the knee is above the face. Breathe evenly; hold for 5 seconds. Repeat on the opposite side. Come back to the center and bring the legs together.

139

Variation 4

Place the right foot in the half lotus posture.

Breathe evenly; hold for 5 seconds.

Repeat with the left leg.

Bring the legs together.

Variation 5

A more advanced way of "going into" the headstand is to raise the hips until the spine is erect. Raise the legs, keeping the knees straight and toes pointed. Lower the legs in the same way.

Stand up very slowly. Remain standing for as long as you held the posture. This allows the blood flow to return to normal.

Lie in the corpse posture, relax completely.

Benefits
- Considered the "King of Asanas" in hatha yoga; it is a panacea for all diseases
- Increases the blood pressure and flow of blood to the brain
- Brings exhilaration of spirit and fills the body with energy
- Is said to increase memory and intelligence
- Variations also stretch the inside thigh muscles
- Variation 5 strengthens the abdominal and lower back muscles

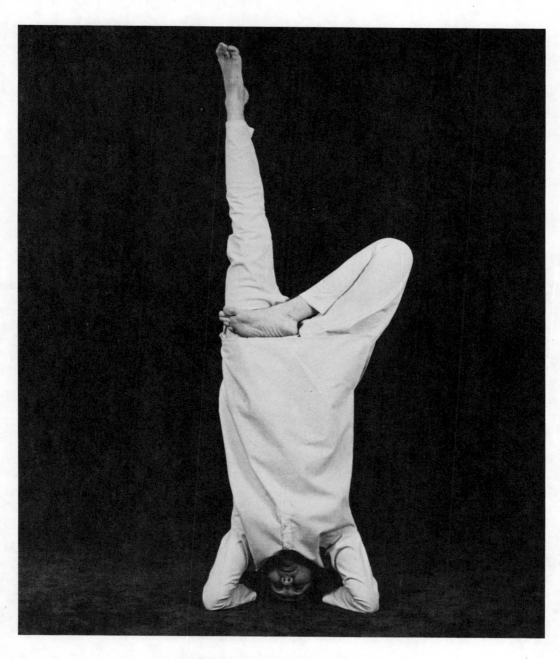

SHIRSHASANA—HEADSTAND
Variation 4

141

RELAXATION

Relaxation Exercises

Following the postures with a relaxation exercise is just as important for intermediate students as it is for beginning students. The first exercise relaxes the skeletal muscles, eliminates any fatigue or strain following the postures, and energizes both the mind and the body. The second exercise relaxes the tendons and ligaments around the joints. During both exercises keep the mind alert and concentrated on your breath as you progressively relax your muscles. The two exercises together should not be practiced for more than 15 minutes.

Exercise 1

Lie in the corpse posture with the eyes gently closed. Inhale and exhale through the nostrils slowly, smoothly, and deeply. There should be no noise, jerks, or pauses in the breath; let the inhalations and exhalations flow naturally without exertion in one continuous movement. Keep the body still.

Mentally travel through the body and relax the top of the head, forehead, eyebrows, space between the eyebrows, eyes, eyelids, cheeks, and nose. Exhale and inhale completely four times.

Relax the mouth, jaw, chin, neck, shoulders, upper arms, lower arms, wrists, hands, fingers, and fingertips. Feel as if you are exhaling from the fingertips, up the arms, shoulders, and face to the nostrils, and inhaling back to the fingertips. Exhale and inhale completely four times.

Relax the fingertips, fingers, hands, wrists, lower arms, upper arms, shoulders, upper back, and chest. Concentrate at the center of the chest, and exhale and inhale completely four times.

Relax the stomach, abdomen, lower back, hips, thighs, knees, calves, ankles, feet, and toes. Exhale as though your whole body is exhaling, and inhale as though your whole body is inhaling. Expel all your tension, worries, and anxieties; inhale vital energy, peace, and relaxation. Exhale and inhale completely four times.

Relax the toes, feet, ankles, calves, thighs, knees, hips, lower back, abdomen, stomach, and chest. Concentrating at the center of the chest, exhale and inhale completely four times.

Relax the upper back, shoulders, upper arms, lower arms, wrists, hands, fingers, and fingertips. Exhale and inhale completely four times.

Relax the fingertips, fingers, hands, wrists, lower arms, upper arms, shoulders, neck, chin, jaw, mouth, and nostrils. Exhale and inhale completely four times.

Relax the cheeks, eyelids, eyes, eyebrows, space between the eyebrows, forehead, and the top of the head. Now, for 30 to 60 seconds, let your mind be aware of the calm and serene flow of the breath . . . let your mind make a gentle, conscious effort to guide your breath so that it remains smooth, calm, and deep, without any noise or jerks.

Exercise 2

Relax the top of the head, forehead, and muscles of the face.

Relax the jaw, the vertebrae of the neck, the shoulder joints, elbows, wrists, and joints of the fingers. Exhale and inhale completely four times.

Relax the joints of the fingers, the wrists, elbows, shoulder joints, and vertebrae of the neck. Continue slowly down the spine relaxing each vertebra.

Relax the hip joints, knees, ankles, and all the joints of the toes. Exhale as though your whole body is exhaling, and inhale as though your whole body is inhaling. Expel all your tension, worries and anxieties; inhale vital energy, peace, and relaxation. Exhale and inhale completely four times.

Relax the joints of the toes, the ankles, knees, and hip joints.

Slowly relax all the vertebrae from the base of the spine to the neck. Relax the shoulder joints, elbows, wrists, and joints of the fingers. Exhale and inhale completely four times.

Relax the joints of the fingers, the wrists, elbows, shoulder joints, the vertebrae of the neck, the jaw, facial muscles, forehead, and the top of the head. Now, for 30 to 60 seconds, let your mind be aware of the calm and serene flow of the breath . . . let your mind make a gentle, conscious effort to guide your breath so that it remains smooth, calm, and deep, without any noise or jerks.

Slowly and gently open your eyes. Stretch the body. Try to maintain this calm, peaceful feeling throughout the day.

SIXTY~ONE POINTS

Sixty~One Points

TECHNIQUE

Lie in *shavasana* (corpse); relax completely for one to two minutes. Bring your attention to the point between the eyebrows and think of the number "1". Keep the attention fixed on that point for one to two seconds. In the same manner, continue concentrating on the points and corresponding numbers through point 31.

Repeat the exercise twice. Practice for seven to ten days. When this exercise can be done without allowing the mind to wander, then continue through all 61 points.

Practice the 61 points exercise after relaxation and before *pranayama*. The exercise may be begun on either the right or left side. But be consistent; if you begin (on the torso) with the right arm, then in the lower extremities, also begin with the right leg. 61 points should not be practiced when you feel sleepy or tired.

31 POINTS

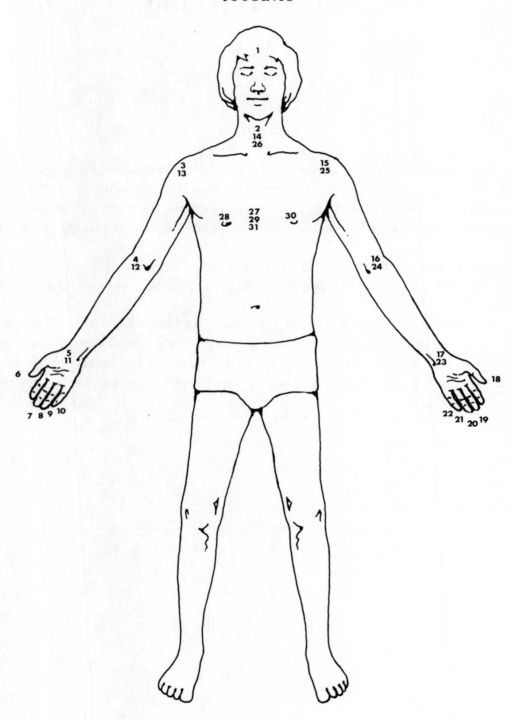

61 POINTS

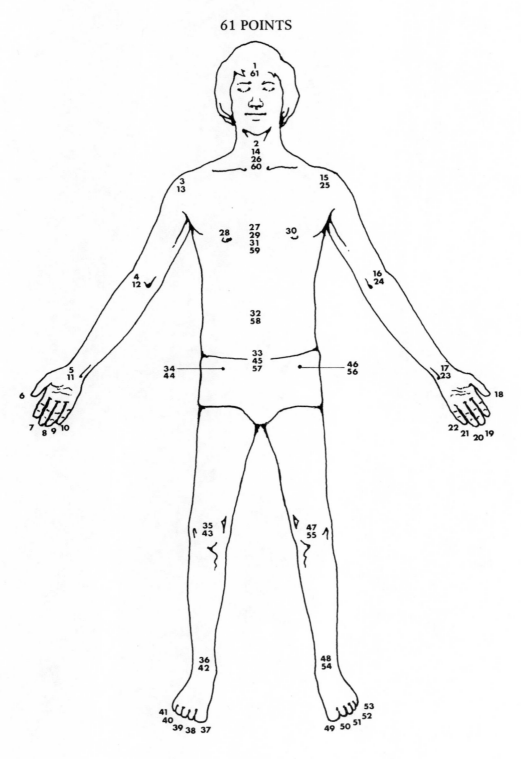

153

PRAṆĀYĀMA

Praṇāyāma

There are a number of *pranayama* exercises which the intermediate student of hatha yoga can practice. If diaphragmatic breathing has become a natural and unconscious function, and the first exercise of *nadi shodhanam* has been practiced for two to three months, then students may practice other exercises.

Kapalabhati, bhastrika and *nadi shodhanam* should be practiced daily. *Nadi shodhanam* can be followed with *ujjayi, sitali, sitkari,* or *bhramari.* These need not be practiced daily, but each should be practiced for some time until they are mastered and their benefits derived. These exercises expand and regulate the motion of the lungs. It is important in all *pranayama* exercises that the head, neck, and trunk remain straight. In *kapalabhati* and *bhastrika* attention is paid to the use of the diaphragm and the abdominal muscles. The chest, shoulders, and facial muscles should remain relaxed. *Mulabandha* (root lock) and *jnana mudra* (finger lock) should be applied with all of the *pranayama* exercises, *vishnu mudra* where specified, and *jihva bandha* (tongue lock) in those exercises where it is possible. The description of active and passive nostrils is repeated because of its importance in practicing both *bhastrika pranayama* and *nadi shodhanam.*

ACTIVE AND PASSIVE NOSTRILS

Usually the breath does not flow equally in both nostrils; one nostril is more blocked than the other. This can be easily observed; gently close one nostril and inhale and exhale rapidly through the open nostril. Then repeat the same on the opposite side. You will find that one nostril flows more freely than the other; this one is the active nostril, the other is the passive nostril. One inhales *prana* through the active nostril and exhales *prana* through the passive nostril. Throughout the day and night the active and passive nostrils alternate. According to yoga science this phenomenon is the result of the alternating flow of subtle energy in the *ida* and *pingala*, the two main energy channels (*nadis*) along the spinal column. For meditation, it is desirable to activate these two *nadis* equally and apply *sushumna* (state of joy in which both nostrils flow freely).

157

KAPALABHATI PRANAYAMA

Literally *kapalabhati* means the *pranayama* which "makes the skull shine." Sit with the head, neck, and trunk in a straight line. Using the diaphragm and the abdominal muscles, forcefully expel the breath. This is followed by a slow, spontaneous inhalation as the abdominal muscles are relaxed. This constitutes one cycle; the cycles are repeated in rapid succession. Begin with seven cycles and slowly increase to twenty-one. This exercise cleans the sinuses and respiratory passages and stimulates the digestive organs.

BHASTRIKA PRANAYAMA

"Bhastra" means bellows. In this exercise the abdominal muscles move forcefully in and out like a blacksmith's bellows. In *bhastrika* both exhalation and inhalation are vigorous and forceful. This constitutes one cycle. The cycles are repeated in rapid succession, again seven to twenty-one times as one's capacity increases. The three variations of *bhastrika* are: front bellows, side to side bellows, and alternate bellows. In all three variations exhalation and inhalation is vigorous and forceful.

Front Bellows—Facing forward repeat 7-21 cycles of *bhastrika*.

Side to Side Bellows—
(1)   Face forward; repeat one cycle of *bhastrika.*
(2)   Turn the head to right if the left nostril is active, or to the left if the right nostril is active. Repeat one cycle.
(3)   Face forward; repeat one cycle.
(4)   Turn the head in opposite direction of (2). Repeat one cycle.
(5)   Face forward; repeat one cycle. Continue repeating these five steps for 7-21 cycles. In this variation of *bhastrika* it is important that the head is completely turned before repeating the cycle. Do not inhale or exhale while the head is turning.

Alternate Nostril Bellows—In alternate nostril bellows, the rapid exhalation-inhalation is done with one nostril at a time.
(1)   Face forward; use *vishnu mudra* to close the passive nostril. Repeat one cycle of *bhastrika.*
(2)   Close the active nostril. Repeat one cycle. Repeat for 7-21 cycles.

The benefits of *bhastrika pranayama* are similar to those of *kapalabhati pranayama*. The forceful exhalation cleans the lungs of the stale residual air which is not achieved in normal breathing. The entire respiratory system is purified and internal vigor aroused. Both *kapalabhati* and *bhastrika* should be practiced in the morning before *nadi shodhanam*.

NADI SHODHANAM

Nadi shodhanam is a simple *pranayama* exercise that purifies the *nadis*. It balances the flow of breath in the nostrils and the flow of subtle energy in the *nadis*. *Nadi shodhanam* should be practiced at least twice a day, in the morning and the evening.

First method
(1) Inhalation and exhalation in all the methods should be of equal duration. Do not force the breath; keep it slow, controlled, and free from sounds and jerks. With practice, gradually lengthen the duration of inhalation and exhalation.
(2) Bring the right hand to the nose, fold the index finger and the middle finger so the right thumb can be used to close the right nostril and the ring finger can be used to close the left nostril *(vishnu mudra)*.
(3) Close the passive nostril and exhale completely through the active nostril.
(4) At the end of exhalation, close the active nostril and inhale through the passive nostril slowly and completely. Inhalation and exhalation should be of equal duration.
(5) Repeat this cycle of exhalation with the active nostril and inhalation with the passive nostril two more times.
(6) At the end of the third inhalation with the passive nostril, exhale completely through the same nostril keeping the active nostril closed with the finger.
(7) At the end of exhalation, close the passive nostril and inhale through the active nostril.
(8) Repeat two more times the cycle of exhalation through the passive nostril and inhalation through the active nostril.

159

(9)   To sum up:

1	Exhale	Active
2	Inhale	Passive
3	Exhale	Active
4	Inhale	Passive
5	Exhale	Active
6	Inhale	Passive
7	Exhale	Passive
8	Inhale	Active
9	Exhale	Passive
10	Inhale	Active
11	Exhale	Passive
12	Inhale	Active

(10)   Place the hands on the knees and exhale and inhale through both nostrils evenly for three complete breaths. This completes ONE cycle of the *nadi shodhanam* exercise.

At the intermediate level students should practice THREE cycles of *nadi shodanam*. Exhale and inhale through both nostrils evenly for three complete breaths between cycles. Either three cycles of the first method, or one each of the three methods can be practiced. Notice that in all three methods the first inhalation is through the passive nostril. The second and third methods are listed below.

Second Method

1	Exhale	Passive
2	Inhale	Passive
3	Exhale	Active
4	Inhale	Active
5	Exhale	Passive
6	Inhale	Passive
7	Exhale	Active
8	Inhale	Active
9	Exhale	Passive
10	Inhale	Passive
11	Exhale	Active
12	Inhale	Active

160

Third Method

1	Exhale	Passive
2	Inhale	Passive
3	Exhale	Passive
4	Inhale	Passive
5	Exhale	Passive
6	Inhale	Passive
7	Exhale	Active
8	Inhale	Active
9	Exhale	Active
10	Inhale	Active
11	Exhale	Active
12	Inhale	Active

UJJAYI PRANAYAMA

Breathe in slowly and deeply through the nostrils. Partially close the glottis so that both the incoming and outgoing air is felt on the roof of the palate. During inhalation mentally repeat the sound So . . . . ooo and during the exhalation mentally repeat Humm . . . mm. The abdomen should be slightly contracted during inhalation. Do not pause between exhalation and inhalation and make a soft, continuous, sobbing sound with the breath. One inhalation and exhalation constitutes one cycle. Repeat the exercise for three to five minutes. *Ujjayi* clears the nasal passages, soothes the nerves, and calms the mind.

BHRAMARI

Inhale completely through both nostrils. Exhaling as in *ujjayi*, produce the humming sound of a bee. Repeat for two to three minutes. *Bhramari* soothes the nerves and calms the mind.

SITALI

Curl the tongue lengthwise until it resembles a tube. Those students who can not do this should practice *sitkari*. Let the tip of the tongue protrude outside the lips. Inhaling make a hissing sound with the breath. Exhale completely through

161

both nostrils. Repeat three times. Many books recommend retaining the breath between inhalation and exhalation in both *sitali* and *sitkari*. We do not recommend it at this stage. *Sitali* cools the body.

SITKARI

Roll the tongue back in *jihva bandha* (tongue lock). Let the lips part, and clench the teeth. Inhaling through the teeth, make a hissing sound with the breath. Exhale completely through both nostrils. Repeat three times. The benefits of *sitkari* are the same as *sitali*.

Index

BOOKS PUBLISHED BY THE HIMALAYAN INSTITUTE

Living with the Himalayan Masters	Swami Rama
Yoga and Psychotherapy	Swami Rama, R. Ballentine, M.D., Swami Ajaya
Science of Breath	Swami Rama, R. Ballentine, M.D., A. Hymes, M.D.
Emotion to Enlightenment	Swami Rama, Swami Ajaya
A Practical Guide to Holistic Health	Swami Rama
Freedom from the Bondage of Karma	Swami Rama
Book of Wisdom	Swami Rama
Lectures on Yoga	Swami Rama
Life Here and Hereafter	Swami Rama
Marriage, Parenthood and Enlightenment	Swami Rama
Meditation in Christianity	Swami Rama, et al.
Superconscious Meditation	Pandit Usharbudh Arya, Ph.D.
Philosophy of Hatha Yoga	Pandit Usharbudh Arya, Ph.D.
Meditation and the Art of Dying	Pandit Usharbudh Arya, Ph.D.
Yoga Psychology	Swami Ajaya
Foundations of Eastern and Western Psychology	Edited by Swami Ajaya
Psychology East and West	Edited by Swami Ajaya
Meditational Therapy	Edited by Swami Ajaya
Diet and Nutrition	Rudolph Ballentine, M.D.
Theory and Practice of Meditation	Edited by Rudolph Ballentine, M.D.
Joints and Glands Exercises	Edited by Rudolph Ballentine, M.D.
Yoga and Christianity	Justin O'Brien, Ph.D.
Faces of Meditation	Himalayan Institute
Inner Paths	Himalayan Institute
Therapeutic Value of Yoga	Himalayan Institute
Art and Science of Meditation	Edited by L. K. Misra, Ph.D.
Swami Rama of the Himalayas	Edited by L. K. Misra, Ph.D.
Science Studies Yoga	James Funderburk, Ph.D.
Homeopathic Remedies	Drs. Anderson, Buegel, Chernin
Hatha Yoga Manual I	Samskrti and Veda
Hatha Yoga Manual II	Samskrti and Judith Franks
Philosophy of Death and Dying	M. V. Kamath
Sanskrit Without Tears	S. N. Agnihotri, Ph.D.
The Practical Vedanta of Swami Rama Tirtha	Edited by Brandt Dayton
The Swami and Sam	Brandt Dayton
Chants from Eternity	Himalayan Institute
Spiritual Diary	Himalayan Institute
Himalayan Mountain Cookery	Martha Ballentine
The Yoga Way Cookbook	Himalayan Institute